Luca Pani

PHARMACEUTICAL RESILIENCE

How to Govern the Evolution of Treatments

CBCO Chief Business and Content Officer: Ludovico Baldessin
Project Manager: Daniela Vidotto

ISBN: 978-88-214-4920-8
eISBN: 978-88-214-4921-5

Luca Pani disclosure: *At present, I am Professor of Psychiatry at the University of Miami, FL, USA; Chief Scientific Officer of EDRA-LSWR, Milan, Italy and of Inpeco SA, Lugano, Switzerland and Executive Director for Global Medical Innovation, NeuroCogClinical Trials, Durham, NC, USA. Observations expressed in this book are personal and they have never been discussed nor have any implications for the Regulatory Agencies for which I worked or with which I collaborated. Especially, any references, even indirect ones, to active principles or possible commercial names of products or pharmaceutical companies are purely illustrative, have an educational purpose and do not imply any support or any assessment of value for that specific product and/or company. Finally, this work has not been economically supported, not even with an unrestricted educational grant, by any pharmaceutical company and/or foundation.*

Edra S.p.A.
Via G. Spadolini 7, 20141 Milano
Tel. 02 881841
www.edizioniedra.it

Printed in Italy
First Published March 2018 Printed by Rotomail Italia S.p.A. - Vignate (MI)

(*) Edra S.p.A. belongs to the LSWR GROUP

Index

Foreword

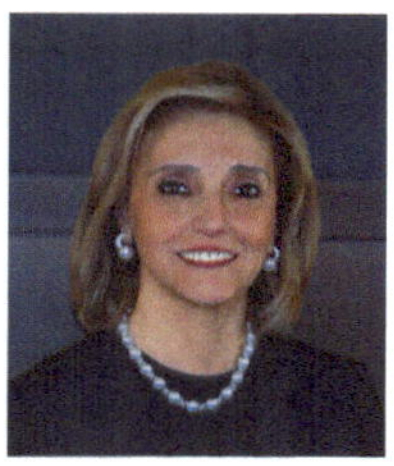

Ornella Barra

The world of health, like many others, is undergoing a significant evolution. Changes are developing at an increasingly fast pace and are having an impact across the board on many spheres of society: economic, institutional, private, ethical, and so on.
There is a tangible sense of urgency and great expectation that affects everyone: patients, healthcare organisations, doctors and companies.
With *Pharmaceutical Resilience*, Luca Pani offers us a compass to orient ourselves in this growing complexity, indicating the cardinal points and helping us find a path to follow.
The special nature of this historic moment is the result of the convergence of at least three macro-phenomena that are becoming evident at a global level, although with noticeable differences in the various areas of the planet: the increase in demand and the growing pressure to which public health budgets are subject; the evolution of the consumer patient; and, finally, the impact of technology.
The demand for health services is continually growing, in both advanced and developing countries, for different demographic reasons. In most developed countries, ageing of the population is now a well-attested fact: by 2020, the number of people aged over 60 years will outnumber children under 5 years for the first time. And although people over 60 made up only 12% of the total in 2015, by 2050 the figure will reach 22%. This means that an increasing number of people will live out their lives with the chronic diseases typical of advanced years and will require adequate care. So it is not surprising that all the major developed economies have for some years forecast an increase in health spending of at least 2–5%[1] by 2040 – probably a conservative estimate.
In parallel, in developing countries, we will see a very welcome increase in the average life expectancy but also an explosion in non-communicable diseases, as widely forecast by the World Health Organization (WHO)[2].
In the face of such a spike in demand, in order to continue to respond to the basic health needs of the global population, health systems must adapt rapidly and find a new centre of balance that guarantees access to treatments and economic sustainability.
According to all the players involved, the direction to take is primarily that of prevention. The health of tomorrow's population largely depends on today's lifestyle, especially among

---

[1] Kibasi et al. (2012).

[2] World Health Organization, *Projection of Mortality and Burden of Disease, 2004-2030.*

new generations. Action must be taken at the cultural level so that it becomes "normal" to conduct one's life in full awareness of the future consequences of the choices made every day, for oneself and for society as a whole. Only in this way will it be possible to change the approach that has been dominant thus far, based on the treatment of diseases. It is here that the second important macro-phenomenon of our time comes into play: the new consumer patient.

Luca Pani shows us how people today have access to much more information and, as a consequence, nurture much greater expectations in terms of access to and quality of treatments. The new habits of acquisition and consumption– in pursuit of fluidity, personalisation and democratisation – also encourage thinking in these terms when it comes to health. The growing awareness of patients must therefore be supported by involving them in the decision-making processes and promoting their empowerment through the very tools of the hyper-technological era in which we live, reaping the undoubted cost-saving opportunities that arise from this. This is a vital provision for re-establishing the system starting from the concept of prevention but also for encouraging a culture based on the overall well-being of the person.

In the last 20 years, technological innovation – the third and last macro-phenomenon – is making its presence felt in almost all the spheres of our lives, including health. As a result of the first applications of artificial intelligence in diagnostics, the creation of databases on organised healthcare and the development of tailor-made pharmaceuticals, we are beginning to witness the extent of this revolution. The digital transformation of the medical sciences is a fascinating area that will bring enormous benefits in the development of more effective and less costly treatment administration methods through which a more efficient system overall can be built. But this prospect still requires a great deal of work and the capacity to govern innovative processes. Before significant improvements in efficiency can become tangible, more time and effort are required by all the players in the distribution chain towards integration and increasingly close collaboration. Above all, it must be remembered that the linchpins of any innovation are people and their ability to generate value through relationships; even in the imminent scenario of e-health, the human relationship will always remain the vital component in any action of prevention, diagnosis and treatment. There are many opportunities awaiting us, therefore, but just as many obstacles to be overcome: from the ethical questions of precision medicine to cultural shifts in vaccines and antibiotics; from the inadequacy of the price-fixing of medicines to the difficulties in the systematic collection and interpretation of precious Big Data; from the waste of resources intended for research to the organisational limits of the existing structures. This book helps us recognise them and learn how to tackle them.

Pharmaceutical Resilience is a glimpse of the near future that awaits us, but also a formidable antidote against the fear of change. The author offers us a solution for every problem, an interpretation, a concrete example to inspire us. Many of these are bound up in Italian experiences, in the many excellent examples of work in the academic, clinical, regulatory and industrial fields of the country – a wealth of knowledge to be cherished and cultivated, with a sense of responsibility, a spirit of adaptation to the international context and a renewed alliance among all the players in the field.

Ornella Barra,
Co-Chief Operating Officer
Walgreens Boots Alliance

1. Recognising change: scenarios that are no longer so futuristic and new/old health emergencies

We live immersed in an ocean of data and information but, paradoxically, we risk being deprived of knowledge and drowning in a sea of ignorance. We must find a way of identifying reliable primary sources in order to counter the "rumours" and discern the really vital elements in the quadrillions[3] of bytes circulating on the information superhighway. This is the real challenge facing healthcare institutions (and not only them) in the years to come. We must be able to recognise quality data, analyse them to convert them into knowledge and, by means of the latter, predict the evolution of the major trends in pharmacology and healthcare in general. This is an increasingly vital in the current panorama, marked by revolutions and paradigm changes that are being pursued at a frenetic pace.
The pages that follow describe a national and international panorama of new trends in pharmacology and of the actions undertaken (also) by the Italian Medicines Agency in order to recognise and intercept them:

- 1.1 World trends in medicine in 2016
- 1.2 The new European Regulation on clinical trials
- 1.3 Sharing clinical trial data: a collective responsibility
- 1.4 International cooperation and new public-private partnerships for research on new medicines
- 1.5 EPSCO conclusions on personalised medicine promotion and focus on the EU dementia emergency
- 1.6 New guidelines published on the EMA website for the development of treatments for Alzheimer-type dementia

[3] The quadrillion is the number that, in Europe, equals a billion billion, that is, a million to the power of four (1,000,000,000,000,000,000,000,000, or 1024). In the United States, on the other hand, a *quadrillion* is a number followed by fifteen zeros (1015). In the United States and the Anglo-Saxon world, the European quadrillion is equal to the *Septillion*, that is, a billion zilllions (109 × 1015 = 1024). Its prefix in the International System is the *yotta*.

1.1 World trends in medicine in 2016

In an issue devoted to the latest developments of 2016, the trade magazine *PharmaVoice* concentrated on the ten major trends that will change the life sciences industry starting from 2016, that is:

I. Precision medicine
II. Patient empowerment
III. Study of the human brain
IV. Cures Act
V. Big Data and analytical marketing
VI. Mobile optimisation
VII. Smart medical technologies
VIII. Reputation management
IX. Healthcare disrupters
X. New health economy

I Precision medicine

Precision medicine attempts to define an approach for the prevention and treatment of diseases that, for each person, takes account of genetic variability, the environment and lifestyle and will enable us the redraw the way in which treatments are developed. In the United Sates, with a relatively limited investment of around US$215 million in President Obama's 2016 budget, the purpose of the Precision Medicine Initiative of the National Institutes of Health (NIH) is to study and develop a new patient-centred research model to try to accelerate biomedical discoveries and provide doctors with new tools and knowledge to identify which treatments work best for the individual person. At the time this book went to press, it was not known whether the amount and objectives of these resources will be confirmed under the administration of President Trump.
In this context, the role of the regulatory agencies in incentivising clinical researchers and pharmaceutical companies to go beyond the model of the so-called blockbuster drugs, ensuring support for the development of solid designs of N-of-1 trials, seems fundamental. In this regard, one of the current regulatory and scientific challenges lies in being able to identify as soon as possible biomarkers that can stratify the patient population according to distinct biological subtypes. This is an undertaking that must certainly involve the patients, as we see later, but also the regulators, the payers, the companies and the academic world,

as well as various European institutions, which have been active for some time. Indeed, recognising the importance of the development of targeted and innovative treatments, and aware that genomic data have become more and more important in assessing the risks and benefits of a medicine, as well as in the control of post-authorisation safety, the European Medicines Agency (EMA), for example, has not only devoted special attention to research into the use of biomarkers in the development of medicines[4] but is also engaged in the definition of scientific guidelines on pharmacogenomics that can encourage the use of genomic data in early diagnosis and the development of personalised treatments. Various national regulatory agencies, including Italy's, for their part provide support and consultancy to the EMA for qualification advice activities on the stratification of instruments and markers to better understand the results of clinical trials. The aim is to verify in advance whether these instruments can ever be accepted and useful in clinical trials and to support the qualification of innovative development methods in research in the pharmaceutical sphere because, in the light of the trends that are already becoming established in modern pharmacological research, this would help enhance innovation in order to offer medicines that are truly more effective.

The other side of this revolution implies, logically, the exclusion – at least temporarily – from clinical trials of all those who do not possess certain biomarkers, making all diseases, once stratified, from a specific point of view, in some way rare, awaiting a treatment dedicated only to a certain subgroup and eliminating all others. In this context and with similar prospects, the ethical aspects of the new research and the development of "selective" medicines at the molecular level must be considered in tandem.

II Patient empowerment

According to the WHO, since 2011 the United States has spent more on healthcare *per capita* (US$8608) and on health as a percentage of their GDP (17.9%) than almost any other country; since then, this trend has remained constant with increasingly high costs. Notwithstanding this investment, the Commonwealth Fund ranked the United States in last place for the quality of healthcare compared with similar countries. It cannot be excluded that the methods by which healthcare is organised in America are at the root of this failure, requiring a rethinking of strategies that put the patients at the centre of the entire preventive-diagnostic-therapeutic process. Patient empowerment therefore represents a change,

[4] http://www.ema.europa.eu/ema/index.jsp?curl=pages/special_topics/general/general_content_000349.jsp.

including in terms of clinical strategies, for the industry because, when individuals take greater control of their health decisions and needs, this inevitably forces the health system to diversify (by definition) and change. For this reason, the industry must move towards the development of strategies that meet the needs and expectations of today's patients.
In the last five years, the Italian Medicines Agency has been very aware of the real patient-centric revolution that is underway and has been working for some time to encourage patient empowerment, providing information and education for the purpose of facilitating participation in the processes of experimentation, development and monitoring of medicines. The Italian Medicines Agency intends to continue to recognise, not just in words, the important role of patients and their representatives in the regulatory sphere, considering it a moral duty to make them an integral and responsible part of the system, informing them about all the aspects that can contribute to improving choices in the healthcare field. In this direction, in 2014, a collaboration agreement was signed between AIFA and EUPATI[5] (European Patients' Academy on Therapeutic Innovation) to boost the awareness of public opinion on the inclusion of patients in the regulatory process.

III Study of the human brain

In recent years, the NIH has announced its second cycle of study bursaries in order to support the objectives of the BRAIN Initiative, which was worth US$85 million in investments for the 2015 tax year. Sixty-seven new awards, totalling more than US$38 million, will go to 131 researchers from 125 Institutes in the United States and in 8 other countries, thereby extending the efforts of the NIH in support of new instruments and technologies for understanding the function of neural circuits and to try to capture a dynamic view of cerebral physiology. Indeed, it is forecast that the global market for diseases of the Central Nervous System will reach US$58.6 billion and will gradually increase starting from 2017. In 2015, US$3.3 billion were invested by companies engaged in the development of medicines for psychiatric illnesses, the highest level of financing in the last ten years. Notwithstanding the terrible stigma surrounding these illnesses and a delay in diagnosis and treatment of psychiatric illnesses throughout the world, various governments have by now acquired knowledge of the social and economic impact of many chronic brain diseases, such as Alzheimer-type dementia; this is probably the reason why we are seeing a constant growth of interest in this sector in both the public and private spheres.

[5] AIFA. "Protocollo d'intesa AIFA-Eupati per l'empowerment dei pazienti" (*Protocol of understanding AIFA-Eupati for the empowerment of patients*), AIFA 2014.

IV Cures Act

In July 2015, almost 350 members of the US House of Representatives voted for the Cures Act of the 21st century, in order to promote development and accelerate the approval of new medicines and devices, especially treatments for cancer and rare diseases. As already mentioned, this measure is consistent with the attempt to put the patient's point of view at the centre in the research, development and widespread use of new medicines, taking account of the advantages that can be triggered by data analyses and by a more rapid and flexible approval process, without departing from the principles of safety and efficacy. In addition to increasing finance for research and promoting the development of innovative treatments available to patients, the Cures Act became law in the United States on 13 December 2016 in order to support efforts in the field of rare diseases and precision medicines and impose new and meaningful prerequisites in the regulation of the technologies of healthcare information and clinical research, as well as various changes regarding the activities of the US Food and Drug Administration (FDA). For example, there is a device that would enable communication between companies and doctors, in accordance with which the FDA should release a guide on the capacity of pharmaceutical companies to provide accurate information about approved medicines that is not misleading and scientifically more rigorous than currently provided. For this reason, in accordance with the typical American rigour and pragmatic vision, the FDA will have at its disposal an additional budget of US$500 million for the next 9 years to implement the law. In contrast, in recent years, Italian regulations have assigned dozens of extra tasks to our national regulatory agency, for the same expenditure, as those who clearly do not completely understand the evolution of the pharmaceutical and regulatory world are keen to affirm. Indeed, these resources, if invested well, can lead to savings, and so the lack of variation in expenditure does not necessarily mean an increase in costs but could also lead to cost reductions.

V Big Data and analytical marketing

The number of digital interactions with doctors, suppliers, payers and patients is increasing rapidly. Since 2017, digital strategies guided by the analysis of human behaviour are increasingly shaping the marketing industry in an even more efficient and profitable way. The intelligent and innovative interrogation of the data already available in abundance from open and legitimate public sources represents the future of marketing, including pharmaceutical. The accessibility of data on consumers/patients, research institutes, institutions and many

private companies, in combination with the instruments that enable all this information to be extracted, analysed and connected through proprietary algorithms of deep learning, will open the path to targeted strategies and effectiveness at levels incomparable with regard to the current ones. The regulatory agencies and the payers, by using Big Data, predictive methods and analysis, can proactively identify the best combinations of messages for both patients and doctors and provide them with more useful information to obtain the best possible results from a treatment, in terms of adherence, follow-up, and short- and long-term results. Moreover, by correlating these enormous quantities of data with the actual behaviour of people as recorded in their everyday lives by portable or perimeter sensors, apps or "intelligent" devices, so-called Data Science will revolutionise the concept of therapeutic efficiency (a combination of the efficacy and safety of a medicine in real life).
These analyses have the capacity to do what individuals cannot do: collect and, above all, interconnect all the available information, instantly suggesting the best means and most suitable and personalised message.

VI Mobile optimisation

This entire revolution would be absolutely impossible without the number of physical users who possess and access communication technologies through mobile and portable devices.

The 2017 global edition of GSMA's Mobile Economy report shows that the target of 5 billion users was exceeded by the middle of 2017, with a forecast increase to 5.7 billion by the end of the decade, when subscribers to mobile telephone services will number almost three quarters of the world's population. The increase in the number of users in this period will firstly be fed by the major Asian markets, such as India, which, according to the forecasts, will contribute 310 million new users by 2020.
Furthermore, the study underscores the transition underway in broadband mobile networks and smartphones, which form the foundation for the 5G era, in addition to the growing weight of the mobile telephone sector in the global economy and in terms of jobs and social development.
While 4G is expanding at a planetary level, 5G is being prepared to supplant it. At the end of 2016, there were 4.8 billion individual users in the world and 7.9 billion SIM connections. More than half of the connections (55%) were on mobile broadband networks (3G/4G), which, according to forecasts, will support almost three quarters of the connections in 2020. The share of 4G connections alone is destined to almost double, increasing from 23% to

41% by the end of the decade, as a consequence of the investments in 4G networks by the operators. At the end of 2016, 4G (LTE) networks numbered 580 in 188 countries, capable of providing 4G coverage to around 60% of the global population.

Looking further ahead, the study forecasts that the first commercial 5G networks (based on LTE version 15) will see the light of day in 2019 and will be accessible to one third of the world's population by 2025. By this date, the number of 5G connections is expected to have reached 1.1 billion[6].

Many of the new users are "millennials", a term that defines – among other characteristics – a population that is never parted from mobile phones. These billions of users, who always remain connected and are part of a world that will see the mobile phone at the centre of marketing strategy plans, are avid searchers and generators of health information as "consumers" of medicine and potential patients.

Whether the end user is a patient or a doctor, the information will be forced to adapt to the flow of decision-making processes and must be available in all formats and easy to use. Faced with increasingly well-informed patients, who directly follow the results of research and communicate among themselves in real time, the marketing model of the future will need to evolve, focusing not so much and not only on brands but rather on clinical outcomes and on greater patient satisfaction, providing solutions through mobile marketing. Apps, for example, may be used as intermediaries between the prescriber and the patient in order to understand the patient's experience of taking a medicine, or to enable the doctor – or the patient – to check the level of availability of certain medicines in a specific pharmacy.

VII Smart medical technologies

According to the results of a recent survey, in 2015, 22% of interviewees used technological methods to view, store and transmit healthcare documentation; in 2013, this figure was 13%. In 2015, the use of technology was greater for people with chronic or severe diseases: 32% compared with 19% in 2013.

It is forecast that progress in information and communication technologies, allied to scientific progress, will significantly change the world and especially the field of health.

[6] https://www.gsma.com/newsroom/press-release/number-of-global-mobile-subscribers-to-surpass-five-billion-this-year.

Huge sums are being invested in emerging technologies in order to provide innovative healthcare solutions, with increasing use of informative sensors, data analysis, bioinformatics and advanced software applications. The result will be a medical and pharmaceutical environment that makes use of "intelligent" technologies in order to improve the decision-making processes in health and the results for patients.

VII Reputation management

Throughout the world, pharmaceutical companies cannot deny that they have a serious social reputation problem, some more than others. In a 2015 survey, only 61% of interviewees said they would be willing to trust a pharmaceutical company. Although this appears to be improving (it was 53% in 2009), and represents the majority of those interviewed, in reality it is a very low number for an industrial sector that has, or at least should have, as its core business the utmost protection of health through the informed use of increasingly effective medicines. American patients assess the corporate reputation of the multinational pharmaceutical industry to be among the lowest of the healthcare sectors, second only to the healthcare insurance sector with a clear profit motive. The results of these surveys are yet more paradoxical when we consider the senseless way in which this industrial division, in its entirety, has literally frittered away its reputational heritage tirelessly built up since the end of the Second World War. The pharmaceutical industry is now called upon, therefore, to demonstrate sincere concern for the individuals they say it wants to treat, by creating a real partnership with patient representative groups, for example, and demonstrating that it is willing to construct a dialogue rather than a business model solely focused on profit.

IX Healthcare disrupters

Faced with the inexorable development of e-health, mobile health and new medical technologies, dozens of companies such as Apple, DuPont, General Electric, Google, IBM and Samsung are entering the generic sector of life sciences in a major way in order to pursue different fields according to their vocation and the skills of their engineers and information technology developers. There are now hundreds of thousands of apps concerned with health: among these, tens of thousands have potential as preventive, predictive, diagnostic, therapeutic and even regulatory aids that can no longer be ignored. The recent news of the agreement between the giant US medicines distributor Walgreens and the PatientsLikeMe organisation, stipulated to be for the purposes of assessing the real-life use of medicines (dosages, safety and therapeutic effectiveness), actually means the creation of a parallel pharmacovigilance network. The warning is clear: official and institutional entities will not be able to ignore this type of initiative and, on the contrary, will have to find ways of collaborating. The entry of technological and engineering companies in the field of medical research is, in general, good news for patients because they can offer new instruments and insights in order to achieve the best therapeutic options. Nevertheless, a century of "regulatory science", for example, in validating the veracity of a marker, must not be lost.

X New Health Economy

The technological progress and empowerment of the patient that we have just described and the increase in health demands from a population undergoing a rapid metamorphosis in social interaction, are the start of a new era in the health sector. In the New Health Economy, "patients" are being transformed into "consumers" who, freely and with responsibility, take decisions, dedicate their time and spend their money in making their own choices – more or less informed, and this may be a problem – including how and when to be treated. The mere collection of data is replaced by the analysis of interconnected information, no longer following the classic model of lines and columns but rather assessing the relationship between entity and attributions in an attempt to anticipate certain events before they occur. Individuals therefore become "co-creators" of the decisions on health, ready to spend more for the tools that, at least in theory, should help them live better. None of this comes free. The earning opportunities in the New Health Economy, now considered the most significant re-engineering that the United States' healthcare system has ever undergone, have already reached nearly US$3 billion[7].

[7] Grom T., Myshko D., Robinson R. (contributions from) "2016 The Year Ahead", *Pharmavoice.com* 2015.

1.2 The new European Regulation on clinical trials

The new European Regulation on clinical trials has been a source of discussion for some years now and we now know the date of effective application of the changes that are keeping debate on the subject alive. So we must be ready for the radical changes that we will have to put into practice from the end of October 2018.

The scenario is forecast to change further after Brexit. Even though Italy is a country of undoubted excellence in the clinical and research field, from an organisational and scientific point of view, it does not manage to exploit all the favourable elements that could make it stand out. Taking account of the fact that, until 2017, England was the leading country for Phase 1 trials, second for Phase 2 and third for Phase 3, it seems clear that Italy should be in a good position, in theory, to become the European hub for clinical research, especially in the field of innovative medicines and advanced therapy, where it has already demonstrated leadership, from both academic and production/industrial points of view and its authoritativeness in scientific evaluation in the role of competent authority. In the same way, in the wake of the international role taken by our regulatory agency from 2011 to 2016, Milan was proposed as a possible headquarters for the EMA, forced unwillingly to move home. The decision was taken a very short time ago. It would have been nice for once to have been wrong about a forecast of this type and to applaud the efficiency of our technical and political system in succeeding in this enterprise that saw us, immediately after Brexit, way ahead of everyone else simply because we had guessed that the result of the British referendum was not at all certain. Unfortunately, that is not how it went and it came down to the drawing of lots, which should simply never have happened[8].

We fear it will take a great deal to reaffirm and reinforce our role in Europe. We certainly need a regulatory agency acting beyond national borders that understands that the regulatory world will be increasingly global and increasingly less open to influence from small, local, political dynamics; we also need an efficient operational infrastructure to reduce the unacceptable bureaucratic delays at the scientific level for a clinical trial, which must, if valid, reach the patients in timely fashion.

The new structure introduced by the European Regulations imposes streamlining of the procedures, greater coordination and unitary management at the national level of the authorisation procedures. We will have a single application presented at a Europe-wide level irrespective of the countries and the sites taking part in an individual trial; the procedure will be managed through a single portal and entered into a single database.

[8] Pani L. "L'Ema giocata a testa o croce: una soluzione infantile e rissosa" (*Ema played heads or tails: an infantile and unruly solution*), Il Mattino 2017;46.

We will work on a single assessment report, almost certainly in English (Brexit notwithstanding!), with a single evaluation team. A completely new development is that, in this team, the presence of a "non-employee" will be mandatory. A patient will make a contribution in terms of the actual significance of the trials. There will be a single tariff and a single informed consent form valid for all Italian patients. And, finally, the results and data of these trials will be open to the public, which will have access to the European database; the sharing and transparency of information for the scientific community and for patients will reach a level never achieved before. Evaluation of the safety of clinical trials will be coordinated at the European level.

Some of this has already happened. For example, in France in January 2016, the network of European regulatory agencies was activated for the purpose of exchanging relevant information and planning appropriate investigative measures after a tragic incident occurred in Rennes during a Phase 1 clinical trial – the first administration in humans – of the molecule BIA 10-2474. One of the volunteers died and three others sustained severe neurological damage. In addition to the inquiries conducted by the judicial authority, two in-depth health service inquiries were carried out to understand how this fatality could have occurred: one conducted by the Temporary Specialist Scientific Committee (CSST) on the inhibitors of the enzyme fatty acid amide hydrolase, set up by the French national agency for the safety of medicines and products for health (ANSM), the other by the General Inspectorate of Social Affairs (IGAS) on the instructions of the French Health Ministry. Both investigations informed all the other regulatory agencies, as far as possible and within the bounds of investigative secrecy, of their conclusions; within a few weeks, ANSM and then the Health Ministry published their final reports.

In the light of the events in Rennes and as predicted in both of the French investigations, the debate on safety matters in clinical trials at the European level has been manifest in a tangible way and, immediately after the publication of the reports, the EMA launched a review of the guidelines containing a description of the data required for first-in-human trials to enable adequate planning and allow them to begin. The review was conducted in collaboration with the European Commission and the member states.

The work of the EMA focused on best practices and guidance with the aim of finding an agreement in the form of a concept paper, published in July 2016[9], that identifies the areas that require change and proposals for further reducing the risk of incidents similar to the French one. The concept paper was used as the basis for a review of the guidelines at the European level in 2017[10]. This process included a targeted dialogue with the stakeholders and public

[9] http://www.ema.europa.eu/docs/en_GB/document_library/Scientific_guideline/2016/07/WC500210825.pdf.

[10] http://www.ema.europa.eu/docs/en_GB/document_library/Scientific_guideline/2016/11/WC500216158.pdf.

consultation on the proposed changes. Two groups of EMA experts proceeded with the preparatory work: one was very appropriately concerned with the pre-clinical aspects and the necessary data from the laboratory tests and trials on animals before safely beginning studies on human beings; the other examined the clinical aspects of planning first-in-human trials and the way these could be improved to protect the safety of participants.
It is perhaps superfluous to point out that clinical trials are essential for the development of medicines and, in the absence of these, patients would not have access to potentially lifesaving new treatments. In Europe, the approval and conduct of clinical trials is currently the responsibility of the individual authorities of member states. The European guidelines therefore serve to ensure that these trials are conducted in the safest way possible and include the necessary prerequisites to collect the greatest quantity of information on a medicine before it is administered to human beings. This is why the level of safety, such that everyone has immediate access to information in a shared way and all the member states together oversee the same trial at the same time, and not individually and at different times as still happens today, will certainly be guaranteed to a greater extent when there is only one dossier to evaluate by identifying those less obvious problems that could slip past unnoticed.

The best-known and most debated aspect of the new regulation concerns the method that will be drawn up in order to have a single evaluation by an ethics committee and – as was predictable – a typically Italian psychodrama erupted on this question. Given that an appropriate law is required and that it will take more than two years to reorganise the ethics committees, reducing the number to around 100 from nearly 300, how much time will it take to adapt to regulations that impose a single national opinion?
Being afraid of change is, of itself, a failure at the outset, and if Italy is incapable of courageously tackling the new challenges that the international context demands, it has no hope of remaining a major player when the change takes effect. Instead, it is vital to work to transfer what can be described as bureaucratic delays to a preliminary planning phase of clinical trials, under the responsibility of the administrations of the trial centres, so that everything is already completed at the time the application for a trial is presented. The aim must be to enable the Italian Medicines Agency, but also the ethics committee, to evaluate the scientific and ethical aspects of the trial, concentrating all the efforts on the effective skills of the regulatory and scientific bodies and not – for example – on the technicalities of insurance contracts. When that occurs, the ethics committees will be able to seize back the role that is their responsibility, that is, to guarantee the ethical conduct of trials, rather than providing support to administrations in handling the bureaucratic aspects of the trial. Whatever organisation we have at the end of 2018, is important to realise that, from now on,

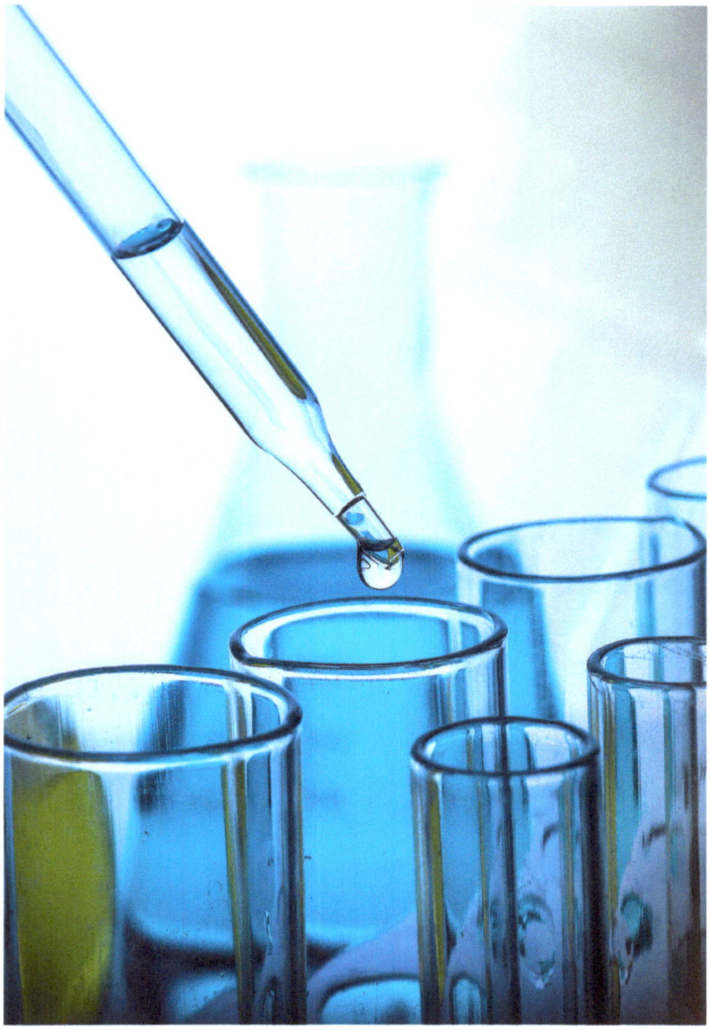

not only is it vital to understand that the role of the ethics committee must change but so must the belief that nothing can ever change. For this reason, the Italian Medicines Agency has already started to work with the ethics committees in evaluating trials presented on a voluntary basis at the European level in a coordinated way among the member states. The pilot VHP project so fervently sought by the Coordination Area for Clinical Trials and by the general management of the Italian Medicines Agency has seen a very high level of participation by the ethics committees and has been a success. All the problems and observations presented about the project were predictable and to be expected when faced with a new model; nevertheless, the number of those who signed up and the liveliness of the discussion confirmed the validity of the initiative. This project will certainly give us important indications about how the clinical trials system may function in Italy.

In 2015, the Italian Medicines Agency demonstrated that Italy is one of the leading countries, taking part in almost 90% of all the voluntary European projects, taking fourth place among the key nations. These data were perhaps not known, even to the sponsors of the trials, but we are proud insofar as we have succeeded thus far, while remaining aware that we can do much more. And we can do still more from 2018, when the new regulations will be applied, but only if the capacity of the ethics committees, and the system generally, is equal to the task, because we cannot proceed at different times or alone. We have the advantage, compared with other European countries, of already knowing the merits and drawbacks of a single IT platform that, from the start – as can be expected in all IT reorganisations – has presented problems but that has also shown the potential to be consolidated and perfected to ensure a platform of interchange at the national level and with the portal already initiated. This is an added value that not all

European countries possess and, in any event, will be very necessary, considering the high number of trials conducted in Italy and the numerous trial centres operating in our country. The clinical trial system is one of the most complex and involves hospitals, universities, treatment and research centres, profit and non-profit making sponsors, ethics committees and competent authorities, together with national health institutes, contract research organisations and personnel dedicated to research. For such a complex system, the organisational simplification introduced by the new regulations can only be beneficial. Scientific training at the highest level and clinical excellence alone are not enough to design and manage a clinical trial, unless the latter is accompanied by sufficient awareness of the rules and regulations of good clinical practice. We cannot do without efficient organisational strategies that also include aspects of budget planning even if, at first sight, that might not come within the expertise of a researcher.

A year may seem like a long time but October 2018 will be at hand in a blink of an eye, and we must be more than ready to seize these opportunities and implement the changes that the new scenario will require in order to reconfirm Italy's role and gain appreciation for our excellence. This is not only for the prestige of the scientific community or the added value of clinical research in matters of investments and healthcare but id also in the interest of patients, for whom clinical research offers the possibility of gaining early access to innovative medicines and hope for treatments that otherwise would be deferred to a time that could, for them, be too late.

1.3 Sharing clinical trial data: a collective responsibility

The debate on the publication of the data on those who take part in clinical trials and on ways of making these data usable and accessible, with respect for privacy and in accordance with defined and unequivocal standards, was recently revisited by the *New England Journal of Medicine*, which dedicated a series of articles to the main focus of all regulatory considerations: the patient.

The patients discussed by the *NEMJ* are increasingly more informed, and, at the same time, willing to contribute and increase their scientific awareness of the medical information that concerns them, because they recognise the value of making clinical data available to the welfare and advantage of many. We are all called upon to respond swiftly to this willingness with the same degree of responsibility, states the International Committee of Medical Journal Editors[11], as did the representatives of the Bill and Melinda Gates Foundation who took part in a meeting of the Multi-Regional Clinical Trials Center of Brigham and Women's Hospital and Harvard University[12] in order to discuss how to make data commonly available, because there can be no hesitation over the need to do so. The mine of information collected in daily clinical practice is recognised as a fundamental resource on which to draw for the benefit and respect of the sick. The greatest value in being able to access the data is the extrapolation of analyses that can generate additional knowledge, that is, important data comes from the patient and must be returned to the patient in the form of an improved level of health.

However, the practical aspects on how to build and manage this immense collection of information are yet clear. One example comes from the Multi-Regional Clinical Trials Center, which has given rise to a non-profit organisation to manage a common platform for the collection of and access to the data from clinical trials: the VivliCentre for Global Clinical Research Data. This is a unique portal that is the prerogative of governments, academia and industry, as well as the non-profit sector, which collects and houses the data, enabling it to be downloaded free of charge through assessment of requests for access conducted by a panel of independent experts.

However, the scenario in which platforms of this type will be transformed into a single vast database into which various datasets flow is still far away. In the meantime, the discussion has shifted to the method of encoding the data to prevent patients' identities becoming known without losing the necessary degree of detail in the information in order to enable

[11] Taichman D.B., Backus J., Baethge C., et al. "Sharing clinical trial data – a proposal from the International Committee of Medical Journal Editors", *N Engl J Med* 2016;374:384-386.

[12] http://mrctcenter.org/projects/vivli/.

appropriate analyses. These considerations are even more relevant when dealing with sensitive data, such as those drawn from mapping the genome, personal devices and sensors and from electronic medical records, which certainly pose the problem of how to encrypt them. Instead of wasting time and resources on seeking to identify complex techniques that make patient data[13] anonymous, with the risk of dissuading patients from sharing them, it would be more appropriate to identify a minimum dataset to be made available free of charge in anonymous form for every trial and thereby enable access to the more complex information only by actively collaborating with and including patients in the complete process, from the definition of the objectives of the trial to the sharing of the results with the research team. The inclusion of the patient in the decision-making processes that concern their health from the very earliest stages of clinical research once again represents the only path to achieve medical science conducted "by patients for patients" in a virtuous cycle where the use of knowledge confirms its central value.

[13] Haug C.J. "From patient to patient – sharing the data from clinical trials", *N Engl J Med* 2016;374:2409-2411.

1.4 International cooperation and new public-private partnerships for research on new medicines

Another problem that has now taken on the nature of a global healthcare emergency was discussed during the WHO's World Health Assembly in 2016 with the announcement of the Global Antibiotic Research and Development (GARD) project, a public-private partnership (PPP) in support of the Global Action Plan on Antimicrobial Resistance with the aim of developing new antibiotics, at the same time promoting their responsible use and ensuring fairness of access through sustainability of the costs.

In addition to bearing witness to the growing awareness in perceiving and tackling the threat of resistance to antimicrobials, the new partnership[14] is an opportunity to reflect on these operating models, known as Product Development Partnerships (PDP), which see the involvement of private actors alongside corporate entities in the research and development of new medicines.

The GARD project is supported by the WHO and the Drugs for Neglected Diseases initiative (DNDi), a non-profit research body made up of five public institutions from various countries, a humanitarian organisation and an international research body.

Since 2003, the project has been working on the development of innovative treatments for the so-called forgotten diseases, such as leishmaniasis, human African trypanosomiasis, Chagas disease and malaria. In this initial phase, the project benefits, among other things, from financing from the Ministries of Health of Germany and the Netherlands, the Medical Research Council of South Africa and the Department for International Development of the United Kingdom. These resources are vital to enable the partnership to properly launch its activities through the planning of the scientific strategy and the identification of other partners to involve, including pharmaceutical and biotechnology companies.

With regard to its structure, GARD is no different from other PDPs, a specific feature in the field of pharmaceutical research and healthcare of the PPPs that first appeared in the 1970s within the framework of the International Cooperation in Development, becoming firmly established in the following decade as one of the most effective instruments to encourage more rapid liberation of emerging countries from situations of endemic poverty through the involvement, alongside public institutions, of the private sector.

According to Michael Reich, professor of International Health Policy at Harvard, these partnerships arose "because neither public nor private organisations could solve the respective problems on their own.

[14] Watts G. "Drug development partnerships look set to grow", *Lancet* 2016;388(10039):16-18.

There was then a realisation," continued Reich, focusing on what happened in the pharmaceutical ecosystem, "by public organisations of the need to involve companies, especially in certain final phases of the development, production and distribution."

Developing medicines for the most widespread diseases in developing countries usually means that pharmaceutical companies receive less remunerative economic returns than investments in research and development of medicines for the treatment of chronic diseases more widespread in other contexts. The involvement of companies, through partnership projects, on the part of public institutions and international bodies therefore becomes fundamental in steering the definition of the priorities for their research and influencing the production decisions, thereby meeting the health needs of the populations of these countries at the same time. The possibility of mobilising additional resources and trying out new business models, of conducting scientific research on innovative projects, limiting the risk by sharing the investments, in addition to the obvious reputational benefits, are some of the advantages for companies signing up to the partnerships, through which the relationship between public and private sectors can develop, ceasing to be defined in terms of conflict but rather a convergence of interest.

Among the most recent successes achieved by the PDPs that deserve mention are the new vaccines for meningitis A and Japanese encephalitis and the combinations of medicines against malaria, particularly suitable for paediatric patients, developed through a project launched in 2002 within the scope of DNDi, which has grown to include a dozen partners, including the WHO and other United Nations agencies, a pharmaceutical company and various academic research institutes.

Still in the initial phase but just as promising is a trial to test the benefits of the use of carbetocin in the prevention of post-partum haemorrhage, which, at the global level, is the main direct cause of maternal mortality, in order to make it accessible to the public health systems of developing countries. So far, the initiative has reached more than 5 million women and is the result of a partnership between the WHO and a pharmaceutical company.

Despite these results, however, as Anurag Mairal of Stanford University believes, the PDPs should not be considered as "a panacea but as a great model, especially for Africa, where the understanding of the market by the global private sector is lower."

To prevent conflicts of interest that could arise between the partners, the identification of a series of realistic and shared objectives, agreed definition of the roles and responsibilities of each partner and the promotion of transparency as the guiding principle of relations between them is vital. This is the reason why – argues Aurelia Nguyen, director of the Policy and market shaping sector of another PDP, known as GAVI, the alliance established to encourage access to vaccinations for children who live in poor countries – "until

the strategy is agreed between the various partners, progress cannot be made. First, a discussion must be made with industry in a deliberate and explicit way on how to align their commercial interests with the public health outcome."
Although the model that inspires the GARD project is not innovative, the new development with regard to existing PDPs, aimed at meeting the health needs of the populations of emerging countries, certainly constitutes an extension of its range of action, also aimed at countries with advanced economies. The repercussions of the absence of new antibiotics under development, for which GARD is trying to find a remedy, are indeed global. The challenge posed by antibiotic resistance could therefore allow PDPs to be unchained from the International Cooperation for Development programmes as an innovative alternative to the established paradigms, exporting this model and scrutinising its effectiveness in other contexts.
Still with the aim of combatting the spread of antibiotic-resistant pathogenic germs, the European Union launched the NewDrugs4BadBugs (ND4BB) research project as early as 2012, which is part of the Innovative Medicines Initiative, a PDP between the European Commission and the federation that represents the interests of the European pharmaceutical industries and associations, the EFPIA (European Federation of Pharmaceutical Industries and Associations). The EFPIA was formed in 2008 as a financing instrument for research activities with the aim of developing new vaccines, medicines and treatments to tackle the increasing changes in the health sector in Europe, at the same time ensuring the international competitiveness of the pharmaceutical industries involved in the programme. Specifically, the aim of the programme is to improve scientific understanding of the mechanisms of antibiotic resistance, the drawing up and implementation of efficient clinical trials and the development of new medicines through the collaboration of public authorities and the academic world, patients, hospitals and industries.
These two partnerships, GARD and ND4BB, institutes for the research and development of new antibiotics, seem therefore able to confirm the forecasts of Reich, according to whom "the complex interactions between national governments and private companies for profitable purposes and all the various organisations in between, due to the kind of things they do and the problems they are trying tackle, are destined to grow."

1.5 EPSCO conclusions on personalised medicine promotion and focus on the EU dementia emergency

That the problems of global public health and healthcare governance have now reached a level of constant political attention is demonstrated by the fact that personalised medicine and dementia were among the topics discussed at the meeting of EPSCO and the EU Council of Ministers on employment, social policy, health and consumers[15], which was conducted in December 2015 at the conclusion of the six-monthly Italian Presidency of the Council of the European Union. In particular, the EPSCO Council focused on a possible definition of personalised medicine within the framework of the context of the European health strategy aimed at the centrality of the patient and on how to improve policies and initiatives at the EU level in order to guarantee dignified living standards and adequate healthcare to people with dementia.

Notwithstanding the fact that everyone has spoken extensively of this for several years and notwithstanding the fact that no commonly accepted definition exists of the term "personalised medicine", EPSCO agreed to describe it as "a medical model that employs the characterisation of the phenotypes and genotypes of individuals (for example, the definition of the molecular profile, biomedical imaging, lifestyle data) in order to draw up in a targeted way the right therapeutic strategy for the right person at the right time and/or for determining the predisposition to the disease and/or to implement swift and targeted prevention. Personalised medicine refers to the broader concept of healthcare oriented to the patient that takes account of the fact that, generally, healthcare systems must be more responsive to the needs of the sick persons."

In acknowledging the coming of the new "-omics" technologies for the development of personalised medicine to offer more targeted treatments, avoiding medical errors and reducing adverse reactions to medicines, the Council identified various challenges that, in effect, undermine the effective application of this new model to current healthcare systems. It is a concern that not all patients have access to innovative and personalised methods of prevention, diagnosis and treatment and that the challenge for member states lies in promoting integration in clinical practice, according to principles of solidarity, universality and equality of access to high-quality healthcare, with full respect for the responsibilities of each state and the sustainability of the individual healthcare systems[16]. Another challenge concerns balanced assessment of the implications, not only of an ethical and social nature but also economic and legal, that the development of personalised medicine implies, with particular reference to

[15] http://www.consilium.europa.eu/it/council-eu/configurations/epsco/.

[16] http://www.consilium.europa.eu/it/meetings/epsco/2015/12/08/.

fixing the prices and reimbursement for new treatments, and to the protection of privacy and the public interest in the treatment of patients' personal data. To this end, among the other recommendations to member states, the EPSCO Council suggests the development of Health Technology Assessment procedures or adjustment of the existing ones in order to assess the impact of personalised medicine in financial terms, taking the patients' point of view into account, among other things, as well as broader cooperation and exchange of good practices.
In the context of demographic change and gradual ageing of the population, EPSCO also identified dementia as a priority for action at all levels in the European context, recognising the significant impact that this disease, and those correlated with it, has on the financial sustainability of healthcare systems. Welcoming the implementation of strategies, action plans and agreed national programmes, it invited member states to reinforce inter-sectorial coordination to tackle the dementia emergency as a single global action, including jointly with the WHO.
Indeed, in the conclusion adopted, the EPSCO Council encouraged the continuation of the profitable cooperation already underway with the WHO and the OSCE and called upon the countries of the Union and the EU Commission to address a series of issues, including:

- The role of prevention, reduction of risk and early diagnosis in contributing to reduction of the costs of dementia.
- The identification of solutions to ensure that prevention, diagnosis, treatment and assistance are coordinated within the countries.
- The promotion of the rights of people with dementia, with particular regard to the ethical dimension of the disease, so that the utmost respect is always paid to the dignity of the patient.
- The exploitation of the potential offered by online healthcare assistance and assistive technologies in order to improve the support and assistance for people with dementia.
- The sharing and availability of existing knowledge on the initiatives underway and their integration in healthcare and daily assistance practice.
- The need to promote the role and continuous training of healthcare operators for the purpose of ensuring the best possible support for people with dementia and their families.
- The promotion of information and cultural education aimed at an improved approach to dementia.

Research must also play a central role. It will be vital to intensify it, starting with the results of the projects financed by the EU (such as the joint screening initiative on neurodegenerative diseases), concentrating in particular on the risk factors and the pathophysiology of dementia and the consequent transfer to clinical practice of effective solutions for managing the disease, and assessing the possibility of partnerships between public institutions, and between public institutions and private organisations.

The protection of mental health is necessary to safeguard public health and the economic development of a country. Other initiatives are the outcome of long processes in which international organisations, civil societies, governments and private companies have taken part. The Global Initiative to Transform Mental Health, for example, is an international alliance that was created with the aim of promoting full participation of people with mental illnesses in the social and economic life of the country, starting with adolescents and the most vulnerable members of society. To this end, the first joint conference was recently held between the World Bank and the WHO with the aim of promoting collaboration between the Ministries of Health and Economy to meet the health and economic challenges that mental health poses.

Moreover, historically, the G7 has always tackled the most demanding challenges of modern society, including those regarding human health, such as the HIV/AIDS emergency, energy investments in Africa or stability in the Middle East. Recently, the G7 tackled the issue of dementia. A key example is G8 Dementia, promoted by David Cameron, then the Prime Minister of the United Kingdom, in December 2013. Following the London summit, public and private investments for research and care for patients with dementia tripled and in May 2017, the WHO issued a declaration that committed all the member states of the who to making dementia a priority.

Therefore, by the end of 2017, it is expected that the Global Initiative to Transform Mental Health will propose that Justin Trudeau, the Prime Minister of Canada, assumes the leadership of a G7 on Mental Health in order to unify the efforts and the international initiatives from all the stakeholders. It is believed that such an undertaking could help support the cause of mental health as a priority for public health and the policies associated with it.

1.6 New guidelines published on the EMA website for the development of treatments for Alzheimer-type dementia

When a pharmaceutical company decides to invest in research and development of new pharmacological treatments for a certain disease, it knows it has to take account of a significant risk of failure. On average, in 96% of cases, the investments bring no return, and the success rate for developing a new antibiotic is 4.6%. However, when taking a gamble on Alzheimer's disease, this probability plunges to around 0.5%[17]. Nevertheless, dementia will be one of the new epidemics of the 21st century. According to the data from the World Alzheimer Report 2015, around 40 million people in the world had some form of dementia and a new diagnosis was made every 3 seconds; the cost of care reached 1% of global GDP and dementia therefore indubitably represents a priority for the world's health systems. In 2016, the numbers increased significantly to 47 million people with dementia, and will stand at 131 million by 2050. The current cost is US$818 billion, which will rise to a trillion dollars (a thousand billion) in 2018.

Despite this escalating emergency, cholinesterase inhibitors and memantine are still the only medicines on the market that can alleviate, probably temporarily, some symptoms of dementia, and since 2002, when the latest drug was approved in Europe, no new medicines have arrived with these therapeutic indications. There being no treatment so far capable of preventing the neurodegenerative process of dementia, the focus is on Alzheimer's disease, the most frequent form of dementia, for which at least the cerebral neuropathological alterations are known (amyloid plaques and tau tangles).

The first attempts to develop vaccines (active immunisation) or monoclonal antibodies (passive immunisation) against certain amyloid protein fragments unfortunately failed, and some researchers believe that, in addition to issues with the structural nature of the molecules, one of the causes of the failure could be the use of treatments too late in the disease when the degenerative process is already at an advanced stage. Others believe, on the contrary, that the entire amyloid theory is fundamentally wrong and responsible for the failures of almost 250 clinical trials and the loss of nearly US$45 billion in investments to support them. Clinical research has therefore tried to generate data in support of the use of biomarkers to enable the visualisation of the amyloid plaques *in vivo* for the purpose of making early diagnoses. The use of biomarkers has shown that the progress of the illness begins in the central nervous system decades before the appearance of the symptoms but does not always develop into some form of dementia (around 30%, which is not a low figure).

[17] Calcoen D., Elias L., Yu X. "What does it take to produce a breakthrough drug?", *Nat Rev Drug Discov* 2015;14(3):161-162.

In addition to the techniques of neuroimaging with radiopharmaceuticals (positron emission tomography), the study of the volume of the hippocampus using magnetic resonance or analysis of the cerebrospinal fluid to study the levels of fragments of amyloid proteins and tau particles should also enable early diagnosis with discrete approximation. Approximation, to be sure, which is precisely why the role of the regulatory agencies appears fundamental.

Patients on whom these so-called disease progression modifier treatments are being tested have been identified by the presence of one or more biomarkers, but with still very slight symptoms, sometimes only an initial memory disorder or no symptoms at all.

The absence of a clear clinical picture makes the diagnosis more uncertain. The regulatory agencies have therefore tried to integrate the most up-to-date scientific knowledge and the need for the development of new medicines to correctly identify the clinical population that could benefit from a new treatment.

If, on the one hand, early diagnosis enables swift intervention in the degenerative process, on the other hand, the uncertainty of the diagnosis means that patients can be incorporated in pivotal trials who have such a slow progression of the disease that it cannot be detected in the short period of a clinical trial (18 months to 2 years).

The certainty of the diagnosis of a model that takes account of the progression time of the disease and the possibility of reliably measuring the results of a clinical trial, even in patients only slightly affected, are among the main regulatory questions to which the new European guidelines (drawn up with a significant contribution from Italy) tried to provide answers. The cultural challenge was to interpret the physiopathological model of the disease in such a way that the regulatory guidelines were effectively based on scientific evidence and were sufficiently flexible to enable adaptation of the processes to new knowledge in a continuously developing scenario.

Alzheimer's dementia is a multifactorial disease. Thus, even though the presence of amyloid plaques and tau tangles is known downstream of the cascade of events that produced them, the physiopathological mechanism that causes their formation is not known, or only partially known.

In particular, it would seem that, in the sporadic (that is, not familial) variant of Alzheimer's disease, there are numerous risk factors (diet, lifestyle, co-morbidity, genetic vulnerability) and physiological pathways (inflammation, insulin resistance, amyloid cascade) that contribute to the symptomatological and neuropathological picture. It is therefore probable that pharmacological intervention in the early phases of the amyloid cascade is the correct approach, but only if the results demonstrate that the accumulation of plaques has effectively been slowed down.

However, it may not be the only approach or perhaps, as the FINGER[18] study suggests, intervention on multiple risk factors at the same time could be more effective. The guidelines also tackled the delicate topic of prevention, for which the data are still anything but robust, but that has steered the pharmaceutical research sector towards new horizons, that of Big Data and Bayesian statistical probability models.
Regulatory agencies like the Italian Medicines Agency have accepted the many challenges of the sector but this is only possible thanks to a broad convergence of all the system's stakeholders with common objectives. Pharmaceutical companies, the regulatory agencies worldwide, payers, the OCSE, WHO and even some governments have found many opportunities for collaboration in recent years. The Workshop[19] organised by the EMA on 24–25 November 2014 or the Integrated Initiative[20] supported by the British Government are two significant examples of the shared desire to arrive at a common vision and to make available the means and knowledge to reach the objective of having new effective and safe treatments for dementia on the market as soon as possible[21].

[18] Ngandu T., Lehtisalo J., Solomon A., et al. "A 2 year multidomain intervention of diet, exercise, cognitive training, and vascular risk monitoring versus control to prevent cognitive decline in at-risk elderly people (FINGER): a randomized controlled trial", *Lancet* 2015;385(9984):2255-2263.
[19] http://www.ema.europa.eu/ema/index.jsp?curl=pages/news_and_events/events/2014/04/event_detail_000932.jsp&mid=WC0b01ac058004d5c3.
[20] Long R. "Finding a path for the cure of dementia. An independent report into an integrated approach to dementia research", 2016. Available at: www.gov.uk/government/publications.
[21] http://www.ema.europa.eu/ema/index.jsp?curl=pages/news_and_events/news/2016/02/news_detail_002463.jsp&mid=WC0b01ac058004d5c1.

2. Vaccines and antibiotics. Primarily a cultural question

If the situation continues as it is, in the very near future, vaccines and antibiotics will no longer guarantee the same extraordinary benefits in the prevention and treatment of diseases, including serious diseases. The unjustified mistrust and disaffection with regard to vaccinations that have forced our government to pass a law in order to increase the number of mandatory vaccinations are seriously undermining the so-called herd immunity in industrialised countries, with the risk of virulent resumption of outbreaks of infections that disappeared long ago or that were thought to have been brought under control. Moreover, the common classes of antibiotics, even some recently discovered, are increasingly less effective in combatting infections as a result of incorrect or indiscriminate use and the consequent growth of bacterial resistance. This means that many infections could once again be feared and that even minor surgical operations may no longer be conducted in safety. There is no doubt – and it is worth repeating it – that the abuse and ill-considered use of antibiotics are the main causes of microbial resistance. Strategies at the global level are pursuing two directions: (1) the promotion of a proper culture on the issue of vaccines and the inappropriate use of medicines in order to combat the disinformation that often leads to falsehoods about the assumed danger of vaccines and to encourage the responsible and appropriate use of antibiotics and adherence to treatments; (2) the research and development of new, increasingly effective vaccines and antibiotics at prices that can be sustained by health systems' budgets. The following pages present a summary of the undertakings in this field implemented by the Italian Medicines Agency, as well as a number of national and international institutions, in the five years from 2011 to 2016.

2.1 Vaccines: victims of their own success

Vaccines are victims of their own success. They have been so effective that they have prevented entire generations from "becoming acquainted" with diseases considered fatal up to a few decades ago, from smallpox to poliomyelitis. When we talk about vaccines, we are referring to one of the most important scientific discoveries in the history of humanity. Vaccines have played a crucial role in extending life expectancy at birth, both for individuals and entire populations, reducing to the maximum the occurrence of many infectious diseases.

After some decades, the success of vaccines turned out to be a double-edged sword, lulling subgroups of populations in industrialised countries into a false sense of security, wrongly believing the danger no longer exists. As queues as much as kilometres long form in the cities and villages of developing countries of people patiently waiting their turn to have their children vaccinated, paradoxically in the industrialised west, anti-vaccination movements, which have even taken root among medium-high socio-economic groups, propagate theories roundly disproven by science, resulting in the return of certain diseases, striking fear and, in some case, becoming lethal.

In our country, we are witnessing the worrying return of diseases that we had laboriously succeeded in eradicating, because the rate of vaccinated individuals is not reaching the percentage threshold that enables the so-called herd immunity. The most recent data on vaccinations disseminated by the Higher Health Institute (*Istituto Superiore di Sanità* or ISS) and published by the Health Ministry show that vaccination coverage in our country is at the safety threshold, a factor that defines a real health emergency. According to ISS, the minimum targets laid down by the National Plan for Prevention by Vaccination have not been reached by any Italian region; on the contrary, there is a diminishing trend in coverage of poliomyelitis, tetanus, diphtheria and hepatitis B, and for measles, mumps and rubella.

The Italian Medicines Agency has always been mindful of these issues and has made pronouncements several times on the importance of immunisation practices and to counter the disinformation, starting from the awareness that vaccination is primarily a cultural concept. In this battle, it is vital to cherish the lessons of the past and to focus on collaboration between all the parties involved: the patients or parents of very small children, healthcare operators, institutions, the academic and regulatory world and industry. Transparent and continual communication regarding the safety of vaccines, above all with the involvement of the healthcare operators, therefore represents a daily challenge and is of fundamental importance in order to re-establish trust in vaccinations.

Aside from the conspiracy theories circulating on the Internet, vaccines are considered one of the safest pharmaceutical products and one of the most controlled, both before and after release onto the market. They are subject to even greater controls than other medicines precisely because they are administered to a "healthy" population who must be reminded that the danger of falling ill is always greater than the very rare adverse reactions to the vaccines. When a person is vaccinated, they do it to protect themselves and others from potentially lethal diseases.

There is a vast body of rigorous scientific literature that reminds us that the most common reactions following vaccination are entirely temporary, last for a maximum of 2–3 days and are manifest as discomfort, fever, swelling, reddening and pain in the area of the injection. Only very rarely do serious reactions occur.

The risks must then be weighed against the benefits. The statistics[22] show, for example, that measles can lead to pneumonia in 1 case in 20, encephalitis in 1 case in 2000 and death in 1 case in 3000. Vaccination against measles[23], on the other hand, can cause severe reactions in 1 case in a million.

Moreover, through the National Pharmacovigilance Network of the Italian Medicines Agency, all the adverse reactions reported are analysed and, in the case of production problems, a temporary block or recall of those batches that turn out not to comply with the standards is put in place.

In the case of vaccines, in particular, we can state that information is the real cure. The Internet is a terrific tool for socialising and sharing data, but it has contributed to the dissemination of pseudoscientific campaigns, especially through informal channels on the social networks that have the sole aim of dissuading parents or elderly people from obtaining the benefits of vaccination. This is an unacceptable trend that the Italian Medicines Agency and other Italian Healthcare institutions do not intend to take lying down. Information, based on scientific evidence, is the only cure for the dissemination of beliefs that are dangerous for the health of the community in which we live.

[22] https://www.cdc.gov/measles/index.html.

[23] https://www.cdc.gov/vaccinesafety/vaccines/mmrv-vaccine.html.

2.2 (Dis)information on vaccines: a challenge to overcome

As we have just seen, vaccines are one of the most important scientific discoveries for humankind, even though they continue to be looked upon with suspicion by some. The impact of vaccinations on the reduction of human mortality is second only to that of water purification, and the prevention of diseases reduces the costs of treatment interventions, making savings in the order of billions of euros possible in countries where the diseases have been brought under control or even eradicated.

The routine immunisation of children is considered one of the most effective actions in the protection of health because, in addition to protecting the individual, it also ensures the so-called herd immunity that protects those who, because they are too young or sick with other diseases, cannot be vaccinated. Yet, for several years, an unjustified and worrying resistance has been encountered among some parents, notwithstanding the fact that the risks from diseases that can be prevented through vaccination are known and notwithstanding the reassurances of the health authorities on the safety and effectiveness of vaccines.

Resistance is largely due to the anti-vaccination campaigns that are rampant on the Web and in magazines and books of no scientific value. These sources of (dis)information cast doubt on the safety and value of vaccinations, especially those for children. Social networks are fertile soil for the uncontrollable exchange of data on health, and it is very difficult for those who have no cultural critical tool to get their bearings among so much information and to distinguish correct information from that created to generate confusion and perhaps advance personal interests that have nothing to do with the health of citizens.

In the United States, a massive communication campaign was conducted recently against vaccination, including on the Web with sites dedicated to the topic, that showed that an increasing number of parents say they are not even ready to guarantee vaccination coverage against measles and whooping cough, thereby exposing their children to serious risks.

In order to combat this disinformation on the Web, a team of researchers at San Diego University conducted an in-depth analysis of 480 websites[24] involved in a campaign of information/communication against vaccination. The picture that emerged is also alarming with regard to the tools of persuasion used to manipulate information and steer users towards other ways of "protecting" health. More specifically, it emerged that, in around two thirds of nearly 500 websites monitored, information and statements could be found on the dangers of vaccines, with a similar percentage placing great stress on the false correlation between autism and the use of vaccines that is regularly repeated.

[24] Moran M.B. "Anti-Vaxx Websites, We're Onto You", *Time* 2016.

On this last aspect, years of rigorous and controlled research have unequivocally demonstrated that there is no scientific evidence to show a correlation between vaccines and autism. Specifically, in more than 15 years of studies, no link has been found between the trivalent measles-mumps-rubella vaccine and disorders on the autism spectrum.

From the analysis, it also emerged that 28% of these sites falsely state that vaccines are ineffective and 43% sound the alarm over the possibility of very severe side effects, such as non-existent cerebral damage. Most of the sites (82%) state that the health authorities do not have the well-being of the population at heart and many encourage mistrust of the institutions by actually suggesting complicity between many doctors and accredited scientists with the pharmaceutical companies. On these websites, it is almost impossible to find balanced content, to judge from the number of the comments posted that are devoid of any scientific rigour by the most virulent anti-vaccination supporters.

In parallel, a much-debated case study was the recent post published by Mark Zuckerberg on his own Facebook profile at the beginning of January 2016 on the imminent vaccination of his two-month old daughter. This message (Doctor's visit – time for vaccines!) was much appreciated by parents and healthcare operators, for making public a choice of a personal nature. Although not explicitly in support of the campaign in favour of vaccinations, the post did encourage parents to vaccinate their children, especially in northern California, which is a real breeding ground for the anti-vaccination movements, and where there has been a significant increase in the occurrence of diseases such as measles and whooping cough. According to a study on Vaccination Coverage Among Children in Kindergarten[25], conducted in 49 US States (plus the District of Columbia), the rate of vaccination coverage in the academic year 2013–2014 was around 95%, and it can be deduced from that figure that most US parents approve of what Zuckerberg and his wife Priscilla Chan did: vaccinated their daughter against diseases.

Nevertheless, immediately after the post was published, on the key sites in the anti-vaccination world, the debate was heated and the founder of Facebook was ridiculed, as was his wife, and accused of putting the life of his daughter in jeopardy with arguments based on junk science and conspiracy theories involving Big Pharma and, of course, the CIA.

The fact that Zuckerberg's post provoked such heated discussions shows how alarming and dangerous the effects of the anti-vaccination movements are; this should not be ignored because, at the level of the protection of public health, all this counts for a lot.

The scientific community must be aware of the messages that reach parents and the

[25] Sether R., Masalovich S., Knighton C.L. et al. "Vaccination coverage among children in kindergarten – United States 2013-2014 school year", *Weekly* 2014;63(41);913-920.

tools and strategies of persuasion used in order to be able to tackle this disinformation and reassure citizens with the force of the scientific evidence and the data that demonstrate unequivocally the safety, effectiveness and quality of vaccines and their importance in the prevention of diseases, including serious ones.

But it is not so simple. Indeed, it has been shown that certain messages in support of vaccinations can have exactly the opposite effect on resistant parents and those who are undecided because their understanding is based on a completely distorted view of reality. The study included almost 1800 parents and led to the emergence of a real "boomerang effect" from the campaigns in support of vaccinations: participants in the study who were sceptical became more so after receiving the information.

So the great challenge ahead is to succeed in combatting the spread of this distrust of vaccinations with authoritative information and communication, founded on scientific evidence and objective data and with appropriate communication strategies and tools.

The Italian Medicines Agency has always been mindful of these issues and has made its views known on the importance of immunisation practices several times, starting from the knowledge that vaccination is primarily a cultural achievement and that it is necessary to be able to communicate the scientific content to an increasingly broad audience of the population in the right way, with follow-up on the results of such campaigns.

2.3 How to tackle the rejection of vaccinations. Choosing between coercion and persuasion?

In recent years, the growing rejection of vaccines and the consequent decline in herd immunity have contributed to numerous outbreaks of infectious diseases, polarising the discussion between supporters and opponents of vaccines.

The advent of the Internet, a multimedia space where, alongside the flow of controlled information based on scientific evidence, opposing views have emerged and coexist without any filter, has exacerbated opposition, which nevertheless has much deeper historic roots. In many cases, this is a revival of past dilemmas, which public decision makers have countered, from time to time, by oscillating between the use of coercive measures and approaches based on persuasion.

The main milestones along this route began with the policy at the beginning of the last century whereby many US states introduced mandatory vaccination against smallpox, both for children and adults, with the imposition of penalties such as exclusion from school of unvaccinated pupils, and fines or quarantine for adults who refused to be vaccinated[26]. The effectiveness of the laws was soon demonstrated; in the areas where such laws were in force, there were fewer outbreaks. The constitutionality of these regulations was also confirmed in numerous legal pronouncements, culminating with that of the Supreme Court in 1905 (Jacobson v. Massachusetts).

The recourse to coercive measures, however – as demonstrated by the controversies, sometimes violent, after approval of the law on mandatory vaccination in Italy – has always raised concerns, because they were interpreted as an intrusion by the state in the sphere of personal freedom, theoretically encroaching on the possibility of choice of parents in the education of their children.

Persuasion became an integral part of health policies starting from 1920, with the appearance and dissemination of modern mass media and advertising. Healthcare operators began to calibrate messages on the importance of immunisation against diphtheria and whooping cough on the basis of the techniques of these emerging sectors.

This practice acquired a scientific rationale in the middle of the century following the development of the vaccine against poliomyelitis, when sociologists, psychologists and other social scientists began to analytically study attitudes, beliefs and social contexts correlated with the various guidelines on vaccination. The efforts of these academics gave experimental

[26] Colgrove J. "Vaccine refusal revisited – the limits of public health persuasion and coercion", *N Engl J Med* 2016;375:1316-1317.

scientific specificity to studies on the reasons people accepted vaccinations or otherwise, both for themselves and their children, thereby making useful tools for developing targeted approaches to increase vaccination coverage available to policy makers and healthcare operators.

We know that the rejection of vaccinations is a heterogeneous phenomenon incorporating a series of attitudes and beliefs, including distrust of doctors and the scientific community and opposition to institutions. However, the reverberations from anti-vaccination theories in the public domain have known highs and lows: times when these theories have been marginalised have alternated with periods in which they have had greater impact, and it would seem that the latter applies today. Improved understanding of these reasons is a fundamental step in drawing up strategies and disseminating more effective messages on the vital importance of vaccinations.

In contrast, many others consider it necessary to reinforce the laws that make vaccinations mandatory, restricting situations in which parents can refuse to vaccinate their children to the point of making exemptions more difficult, following the example of California, the third US State to have eliminated the legitimisation of non-scientific reasons for refusal in 2015, or Italy, where a law has just been approved by parliament. This law has "permanently" made the following vaccinations mandatory: those against polio, diphtheria, tetanus, viral hepatitis B, whooping cough, and type B *haemophilus influenzae*. Of course, this law is entirely reasonable but it is difficult to understand why four vaccinations remain optional "until a subsequent different evaluation" after a three-year verification period, that is, until 2020. These four vaccinations are those against rubella, mumps, chickenpox but, above all, measles, the importance of which can easily be deduced from the severity of the complications of this disease, the worrying fall in vaccination coverage and the consequent vertiginous increase in the number of cases in Italy.

As usual, we never succeed in going all the way, not even when doing the right things.

Undoubtedly, a persuasive strategy would be ethically and politically more acceptable although it would require much more time and a decidedly greater intensity of work. Persuasion and coercion can nevertheless be considered necessary and coessential. No strategy that relies only on one or the other would be entirely effective. The combination of the two approaches is therefore the greatest challenge facing public decision makers on vaccinations; in order to balance and bring together effectiveness, efficiency, ethics and political acceptability, they must all be incorporated in a single strategy[26].

2.4 Immunisation strategies and the importance of defining a sustainable price for vaccines

Great successes in the history of medicine have been possible thanks to vaccines: smallpox has been eradicated, poliomyelitis is largely under control and the incidence of typical childhood diseases, such as measles and rubella, has been greatly reduced where there is adequate vaccination coverage (>90%). Bacterial meningitis is becoming rare in the countries that vaccinate their children. It is possible to prevent hepatitis A and B and vaccination is spreading against infection with rotavirus, the main viral cause of death by diarrhoea and infantile dehydration in the world and, in particular, in developing countries but not, it must be said, in industrialised countries where the complications can be controlled through hospitalisation. Various forms of cancer caused by viruses can now be prevented. All this and much more is due to the dissemination of vaccines, especially in the last 50 years.

Immunisation is universally considered to be a cost-effective public health intervention, however the cost/benefit ratio, and therefore interest in promoting its widespread use, varies depending on a number of factors, including the epidemiology of the disease, its severity and the alarm that an epidemic creates among the population; moreover, the advantage of investing in immunisation is greater in countries that spend more on treating those diseases that can be prevented with vaccines. Cost/benefit assessments have an increasing impact on current health policies, which have to juggle with the ethical imperative of ensuring an optimal level of healthcare while reducing expenditure on high-cost interventions with limited benefits. Moreover, the field of research into vaccines presents a high degree of risk, both for the companies engaged in their development and for those who have to finance these kinds of studies. The process between the discovery and authorisation of a new vaccine requires a lot of time and huge investments, with a high failure rate. According to some estimates, only one in ten candidate vaccines reaches the goal of approval after completing all the experimental tests and overcoming the numerous industrial production problems; the time and cost of the entire process range from 10 to 15 years and more than a billion dollars, respectively[27].

This gives rise to the need to reconcile immunisation policies with fair profits for the industry that are sustainable for public budgets. We devoted the preceding volume in this series to this issue (Luca Pani, *Sustainable Innovation*) and, specifically, we found an interesting editorial on

[27] *PhRMA Vaccine Fact Book* 2013; http://www.phrma.org/resources/resource-library#All.

vaccines published in *JAMA* by H.C. Meissner of Tufts University School of Medicine of Boston[28]. The need for greater transparency on the prices and costs of development of vaccines requires guidelines or clearer recommendations on the use of new vaccines and agreement over decisions on the development objectives among health authorities, including the regulatory agencies, such as the Italian Medicines Agency who are also payers, and producers.

Given that new increasingly costly vaccines are in development or are being considered for inclusion in the immunisation programmes for children, pregnant women and the elderly population, the effectiveness, safety, burden of the disease, fairness and compatibility with existing vaccination programmes will become increasingly relevant issues.

In the not too distant future, vaccines could be available against pathogenic agents, and consensus on the use of a specific vaccine will not be easy to reach. Costs will have an impact on the recommendations. It will not be simple to find a balance between the efforts to contain prices and the need to incentivise the development of new vaccines. Establishing a model of price definition will be fundamental to ensure broad access to the significant advantages that future vaccines will certainly provide.

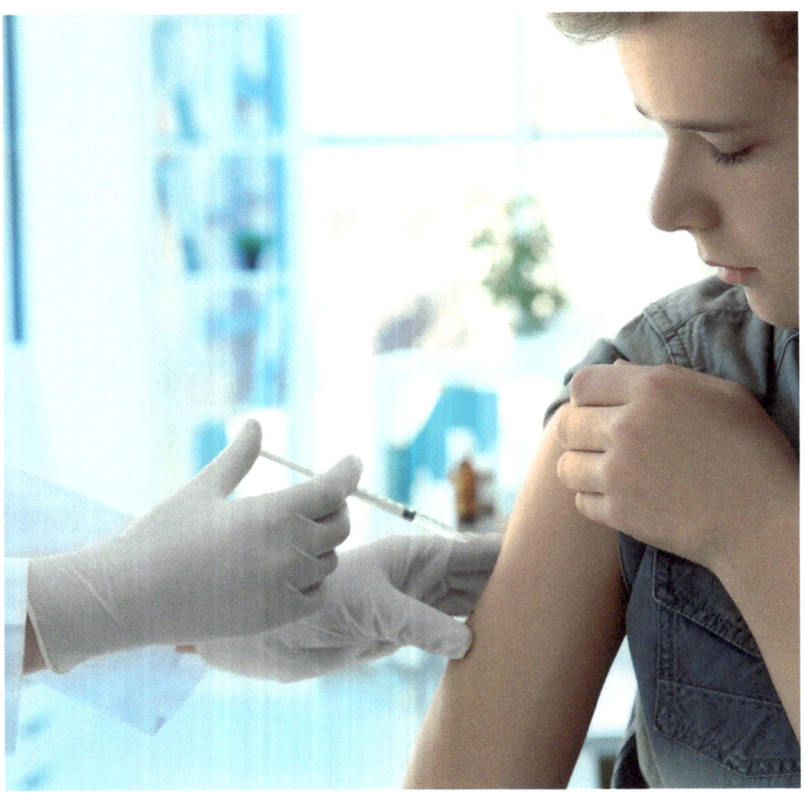

Moreover, it is from this area of research that significant responses to as yet unsatisfied health needs are expected in the coming years and not only in the field of infectious diseases. The extraordinary technological advances in digitised knowledge of the genome gives hope that therapeutic and preventive vaccines for cancer can soon be perfected and, further into the future, for Alzheimer's disease, autoimmune diseases, and even for dependence on narcotics.

[28] Meissner H.C. "Immunization policy and the importance of sustainable vaccine pricing.", *JAMA* 2016;315(10):981-982.

This is a fascinating scenario that brings with it the dilemma of sustainability for public health systems. A key aspect will be to define the research objectives and early agreement on vaccine development programmes among producers, regulators and the Health Technology Assessment Bodies. This is exactly what the Italian Medicines Agency has done in the last 5 years with the national scientific advice and its active role at the heart of the European Agency in the parallel HTA/EMA procedures, which has enabled the input of the regulatory authorities and the HTA bodies of various European countries to be obtained at the same time. In recent years, the expertise acquired by the Agency has enabled the field of HTA evaluation to be extended to seasonal influenza vaccines and to the first "quadrivalent" influenza vaccines, as well as collaboration with the WHO in the evaluation of vaccines for poliomyelitis, diphtheria, tetanus and type B *haemophilus influenzae*.
In consideration of the complexity of new vaccines and their potential impact across an increasingly broad spectrum of diseases with different prevalence, epidemiology and repercussions on health depending on the geographic area and the country involved, it is also fundamental to define at the national level the priorities and prerequisites for the allocation of resources by adopting new strategies of pharmacological and economic evaluation and testing for authorisation and price negotiation models for vaccines as already used successfully by the Italian Medicines Agency for other very high-cost medicines.

2.5 Antimicrobial resistance: how to tackle a global threat

A "post-antibiotic era" is an apocalyptic scenario in which theoretically mundane infections, if an infection can ever be considered as such, evade the weapons of modern medicine and become untreatable, taking the world back, from a health point of view, to the millennia before the Second World War. This is now a real threat for global public health, as stated many times by the WHO and European and Italian institutions. Such a state of affairs is emerging rapidly and simultaneously throughout the world due, mainly, to the excessive and inappropriate use of antibiotics, both for human and veterinary use.

The scientific community and many institutions assigned to the protection of health have raised the alarm on the development of antimicrobials for a long time in the face of still rather limited public perception, including on the part of doctors and veterinary surgeons, of the phenomenon at a global level.

The Italian Medicines Agency has been engaged for years on this front and since 2008 it has conducted a multimedia communication campaign, renewed annually, with the aim of reminding the general population and healthcare operators to "defend our defences" and to use antibiotics in accordance with very specific rules[29].

Since the early months of 2012, the Italian Medicines Agency's commitment has not been limited to this communication campaign but continues every day by issuing information of a regulatory nature[30] to a list of around 190,000 contacts, most of whom are doctors and healthcare operators. In recent years, hundreds of bulletins have also been published on this matter on the Italian Medicines Agency's portal, often picked up by the media, in an attempt to disseminate greater awareness about a problem that knows no barriers.

Data collected by the Agency's Monitoring Centre on the use of medicines (OsMed) confirm a reduction in expenditure and registered consumption for this category. Limiting the analysis to the five-year period 2010–2015, it can be seen that, in 2010, the expenditure was € 14.5 per head, whereas in 2015 it fell to € 10.8, with an average annual variation of –5.7%.

In the same period, consumption also decreased. In 2010, 24.6 doses of antibiotics were administered by the National Health Service to every 1000 inhabitants, falling to 23 doses in 2015. The average annual variation in consumption was –1.3%. In 2016, antimicrobial medicines were the second highest category of public expenditure for medicines (€ 72.5 per head). A net difference was revealed between NHS healthcare (expenditure reduced by

[29] AIFA. "Senza regole gli Antibiotici non funzionano. Campagna AIFA sul corretto uso degli Antibiotici (2014-2015)" [*Without rules, Antibiotics don't work.* AIFA campaign on the correct use of Antibiotics (2014-2015)]. AIFA.

[30] AIFA. "Pillole dal Mondo" [*Pills from the World*]. http://www.aifa.gov.it/content/pillole-dal-mondo-0.

5.2% compared with 2015) and hospital use (an increase of 9.5% compared with 2015)[31]. These numbers indicate a positive trend but are certainly not sufficient. One of the most age-old problems is certainly the "north-south divide" whereby southern regions consume a significantly higher number of doses, without any justification from an epidemiological point of view. The regional variability highlights areas of excellence, such as Liguria (16.2 daily doses for every 1000 inhabitants) and the Autonomous Province of Bolzano (14.4 daily doses for every 1000 inhabitants), and frankly unacceptable and inexplicable situations such as Campania (32.27 daily doses/1000 inhabitants per day), Apulia (30.3 daily doses/1000 inhabitants per day) and Calabria (28.4 daily doses/1000 inhabitants per day).

The Agency's approach in 2011–2016 was to favour an overall view of the problem and to emphasise the best practices in those few regions with the best performances (e.g. Emilia Romagna, which created working groups focused on the implementation of specific guidelines, such as the publications "Acute otitis media in paediatric age"[32] and "Pharyngotonsillitis in paediatric age"[33]), in order to make them available to the regions with decidedly less gratifying data.

The Italian Medicines Agency then actively took part in the working group set up by the Health Ministry to draw up a national plan to combat microbial resistance, and were involved in the European and international working groups through the contribution of its experts.

At the European level, evaluation of the experiences of countries where lower consumption of antibiotics are recorded is of particular interest. The Netherlands is the most virtuous European country, as a result of a different system of packaging medicines that enables unitary doses and personalised packages to be prepared.

The ARNA study, financed by the European Union and conducted by a team of Dutch researchers, concluded that one of the main causes of the phenomenon of self-medication with antibiotics is leftovers, that is, when doses exceed the number prescribed by GPs and a surplus remains available to the patients. The study conducted a survey in seven European countries, including Italy; of 9313 Italian patients interviewed, 9% said they used antibiotics without a medical prescription and, of these, 87% used the remains of packets of antibiotics available within the family and from relatives. In the light of these findings, our country should also set limits on the prescription of antibiotics in the sphere of individual treatment but, clearly, all this cannot be solved by some newspaper headline or in some blog that refers

[31] Magnano R. "Rapporto Osmed 2016: spesa farmaceutica totale a +1,6%. Antibiotici ancora in salita. Melazzini (AIFA): «Grande impegno sull'innovazione»" (*Osmed Report 2016: total pharmaceutical expenditure at +1.6%. Antibiotics still on the rise. Melazzini (AIFA): "Major undertaking on innovation*). *Sanità24* 2017.

[32] http://assr.regione.emilia-romagna.it/it/servizi/pubblicazioni/rapporti-documenti/oma-guida-rapida-2015.

[33] http://assr.regione.emilia-romagna.it/it/servizi/pubblicazioni/rapporti-documenti/faringotonsillite-guida-rapida-2015.

to the famous "single packet" without implementing regulations that rethink the feasibility of similar worthy measures and, above all, individuals taking responsibility.
A Eurobarometer survey commissioned by the European Commission also brought to light the lack of awareness of the effects arising from the use of antimicrobials (antibiotics in particular), especially when inappropriate. According to the survey, more than a third of Europeans took antibiotics in the 12 months before the survey, but, at the same time, the results showed that knowledge of the mechanism of action of these medicines remains low. It is indicative that 57% of Europeans do not know that antibiotics are ineffective against viruses. According to a statement from the European Commission, the results of the survey clearly demonstrate the existence of a direct link between better information and lower consumption.
In Italy, 43% of those interviewed stated that they had taken an antibiotic in the previous 12 months and, in 94% of cases, the antibiotic was obtained "from a doctor".
Moreover, it is the author's personal experience, anecdotal and so with no scientific value, that a prominent GP in the Capital "used to prescribe" an antibiotic by telephone for a lady with a sore throat in the month of July "caused by the air-conditioning" – such was the diagnosis – without even visiting her or even a reported rise in her temperature. It is not surprising, then, under these conditions, that understanding in our country of the action mechanisms of these medicines is still poor, with 60% of those interviewed convinced that "antibiotics kill viruses" and 38% sure that they were "effective against colds and 'flu". Twenty-one percent of the sample were convinced that treatment with antibiotics could be stopped "when you feel better".
The Eurobarometer data confirm what is reported by the Italian Healthcare institutions, that is, the existence of cultural problem in the approach to this extraordinary class of medicines, which requires targeted and synergic interventions with the involvement of all the actors in the health system. The appropriateness of prescription is influenced by numerous factors and, in the case of antibiotics, they are undoubtedly being used excessively without any therapeutic necessity.
The Commission's Action Plan on AMR (2011–2016), currently being evaluated, will contribute, together with the Eurobarometer results, to the work to identify the added value of specific actions by the EU in the fight against antimicrobial resistance. The aim is to continue to ensure that the EU is a leading region for the adoption of best practices in the field of microbial resistance, providing an important boost to innovation and research in the development of new antibiotics and identifying valid therapeutic alternatives to these medicines. We are clearly guilty of not having invested significant public resources in refresher courses for all those prescribing doctors whose inadequate approaches must have

cost our health service a great deal and had a major effect on the health of patients. For this reason, the Italian Medicines Agency has continued with the annual campaigns to make citizens and healthcare operators aware of the importance of using antibiotics only when necessary and with a prescription from a doctor who is certain of their actual usefulness, of never interrupting treatment before the time indicated by the doctor or, in any event, only on his advice, and not taking antibiotics to treat viral infections.

In recent years the Agency has devoted more resources to this issue than to other therapeutic areas that also present critical problems to try and combat the real health emergency of antibiotic resistance. We hope these efforts continue into the future, replicating the initiatives that have enabled the national picture to be improved overall and implementing new ones, involving all the local organisations. Only through a unitary and community-oriented NHS will it be possible to achieve objectives that concern the health of everyone, defeating the invisible enemies, such as microorganisms, that know no bounds.

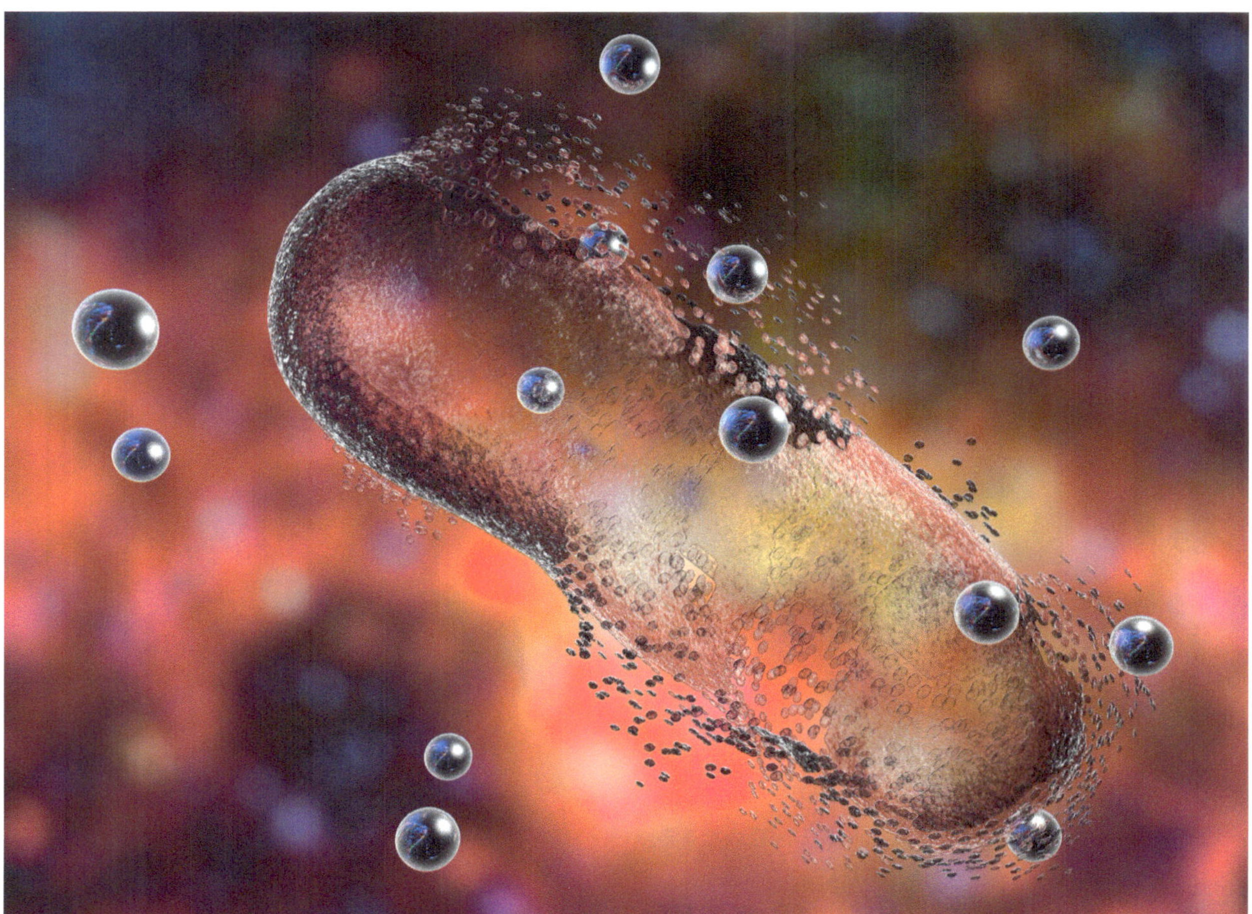

2.6 Antibiotic resistance: a global risk that requires shared strategies

"The danger to human health from antibiotic resistance is much more worrying than the financial meltdown of 2008"[34], this is the argument put forward by Jim O'Neill, an economist, former Chairman of Goldman Sachs and former British Trade Minister, commissioned by the British Government to analyse the problem of antibiotic resistance and to propose reliable solutions on a global scale.

As also reported in the *Economist*[35], the Review on Antimicrobial Resistance (AMR) headed by Lord O'Neill estimated that bacterial infections will cause around 10 million deaths a year in the world in 2050, far exceeding deaths from cancer (8.2 million), diabetes (1.5 million) or road accidents (1.2 million) with costs estimated to be in excess of US$100 trillion.

Antibiotics are a vital tool in combatting various types of infection, as illustrated by the fact that surgical operations, simple or complex, could never be carried out, even with all today's asepsis procedures, without the aid of these medicines. For this reason, excessive and inappropriate use, which allows the development of "resistant" bacteria, limits their effectiveness, creating one of the most serious threats to public health that the institutions have ever been called upon to tackle.

In Europe, 4 million infections occur every year from antibiotic-resistant germs, causing more than 37,000 deaths[36] and using significant resources (health and otherwise) amounting to around € 1.5 billion a year[37]; in the United States, 2 million people have been affected by an infection resistant to antibiotics with around 50,000 deaths and expenditure of more than € 20 million[34].

In Italy, resistance to antibiotics remains one of the highest in Europe and, in most cases, is above the European average. Every year in our country, between 7% and 10% of patients face a multiresistant bacterial infection with thousands of deaths. Infections correlated with healthcare strike around 284,100 patients every year, causing between 4500 and 7000 deaths a year. At the international level, the consensus of the scientific community identifies two main approaches on which to act: the first is an immediate and profound cultural change in the population and in the medical and veterinary community that leads to truly appropriate use of antibiotics in such a way as to reduce their misuse and extend their therapeutic effectiveness for as long as possible.

---

[34] *The Review On Antimicrobial Resistance*, Chaired By O'Neill J., "Tackling Drug-resistant Infections globally: Final Report and Recommendation", 2016.

[35] https://www.economist.com/news/leaders/21699116-how-combat-dangerous-rise-antibiotic-resistance-when-drugs-donu2019t-work.

[36] ECDC – European Centre for Disease Prevention and Control.

[37] WHO – World Health Organization.

The second is a long-term strategy that emphasises the promotion of incentives for the introduction of innovative treatments able to tackle resistant strains. A good example comes from the United States where the Obama Government (in this case also, we do not know what President Trump will do) extended the use of funds earmarked for bioterrorism to the development of antibiotics active against high-resistance microorganisms, allocating around US$1.2 billion in 2016 alone[38]. At the same time, the Infectious Diseases Society of America (IDSA) launched the "10 × '20"[39] initiative for the purpose of creating ten advanced antibiotics by 2020; currently, seven medicines are under trial.
Among the various solutions identified by the British Review on AMR, is a recommendation that a Global Innovation Fund of US$2 billion should be established to finance research in the initial phase and the introduction of a pay or play system, which imposes additional financial charges on those companies that decide not to invest in research and development of new antibiotics. For companies that decide to "play", on the other hand, a "return" of US$1–1.5 billion is envisaged for any new antimicrobial medicines successfully brought to market.
Moreover, a British economist encourages governments to promote financial incentives for the development of new diagnostic tests that can avoid the pointless administration of antibiotics. If doctors or pharmacists could instantly find out, with a cheap kit, for example, whether an infection is viral or bacterial, many inappropriate prescriptions could be avoided. In the same way, the development of tools designed to favour the identification of the most suitable antibiotics for eradicating an infection would succeed in reducing the emergence of resistant strains.
The importance of vaccines is also underlined in the report. The use of vaccines would also reduce the need to use antibiotics. Vaccines can combat resistance to medicines because they reduce the number of cases of infection and the need to resort to antibiotics. For example, vaccines that protect from the bacteria that cause pneumonia, *Streptococcus pneumoniae*, should be administered worldwide. A "universal coverage with an anti-pneumococcal conjugate vaccine, which has already been used in various parts of the world, could prevent around 800,000 deaths a year among children under 5 caused by the *Streptococcus pneumoniae* and could also prevent more than 11 million days of antibiotic use in these children, reducing the probability of resistance developing."
The problem of microbial resistance does not have a single solution and must therefore be combatted on various fronts; a joint effort is necessary by institutions at the international level that requires not only policies aimed at promoting the development of new medicines

[38] https://obamawhitehouse.archives.gov/sites/default/files/docs/national_action_plan_for_combating_antibotic-resistant_bacteria.pdf.
[39] http://www.idsociety.org/10x20/.

but, above all, intense activity to make the population aware; the commitment of healthcare operators is required so that responsible management of antibiotic prescriptions is disseminated and consolidated.

As we have said, since 2008, the Italian Medicines Agency has been engaged in the promotion of the correct use of antibiotics through widespread and dedicated communication campaigns, encouraging patients not to take this class of medicines in order to cure influenza, viral infections or colds of non-bacterial origin but to resort to antibiotics only when necessary and on prescription by a doctor, scrupulously following the doses and times of treatment in order not to undermine its effects.

Using antibiotics well is a responsibility of the individual with regard to their own health so that they always have effective medicines available for their disease, and it is also a collective responsibility. Not doing so encourages the development of resistance that puts the health of the community seriously at risk.

2.7 Being born in the era of antibiotic resistance

The issue of antibiotic resistance, especially with its repercussions at the early phases of the life of newborns, was at the centre of a recent article published on the WHO website by Anthony Costello, WHO Director of Maternal, Infantile and Adolescent Health, and Stefan S. Peterson, UNICEF's Health Manager.

According to the two authors, maternal and neonatal mortality is not confined to the past. Overall, regarding infections alone, incredibly, 30,000 mothers and 400,000 newborns die per year, mostly in poor countries. Restricting the data to the largest hospitals – where bacteria have a greater probability of developing resistance to antibiotics – some studies show that around 40% of infections in newborns are resistant to standard treatments. Newborns, especially if born prematurely, do not have a fully developed immune system and that is why they are more exposed to infections spread in hospitals and bacterial diseases from their mother. The risks obviously increase when the health facilities lack hygiene services, running water and other basic sanitary conditions, as often happens in developing countries, where not infrequently the implementation of effective strategies to combat infections is obstructed by chronic difficulties in accessing antibiotics.

The situation seen in rich countries is different, indeed diametrically opposite; maternal and infantile mortality is now rare, following a century of constant improvements in hygiene and infection control. Mortality rates fell, for example, after 1934 with the availability of antibacterial sulphonamides for the rapid treatment of infections. It was precisely the efficacy of antibiotics, however, that led many healthcare operators to increasingly prescribe them, even when not necessary, e.g. against viral diseases, generating irresponsible excess use of antibiotics, with the appearance of increasingly resistant bacteria and the gradual loss of efficacy of the antibiotics currently available.

Protecting the life and health of mothers and newborns therefore requires strategies and interventions at the global level aimed at rebalancing the existing inequality of access, on the one hand, and excess consumption of antibiotics, on the other, throughout the planet. The first step indicated by the authors is obviously to stop the spread of infections in order to avert recourse to antibiotics. To this end, it is vital that all health facilities have access to running water and clean toilets, and that healthcare operators follow good hygiene practices, such as washing their hands frequently.

Moreover, policies must also be implemented to reduce hospital stays. Discharge of mothers and newborns as early as possible will minimise the risk of exposure to hospital bacteria. Mothers must be educated about the importance of breast-feeding to reinforce the immune system of newborns.

Finally, before administering antibiotics, doctors should be obliged to check whether they are really necessary and to prescribe responsible doses.
With the growing awareness that is developing about these problems, attention is drawn to initiatives such as the adoption by the World Health Assembly, the decision-making body of the WHO, of a global action plan to tackle antimicrobial resistance, aimed at encouraging practices to reduce infections and optimising the use of the antibiotics already available, as well as encouraging the development of new ones. Antibiotic resistance was also discussed during the G20 summit in China in September 2016 and will be the subject of a meeting of the General Assembly of the United Nations[40].

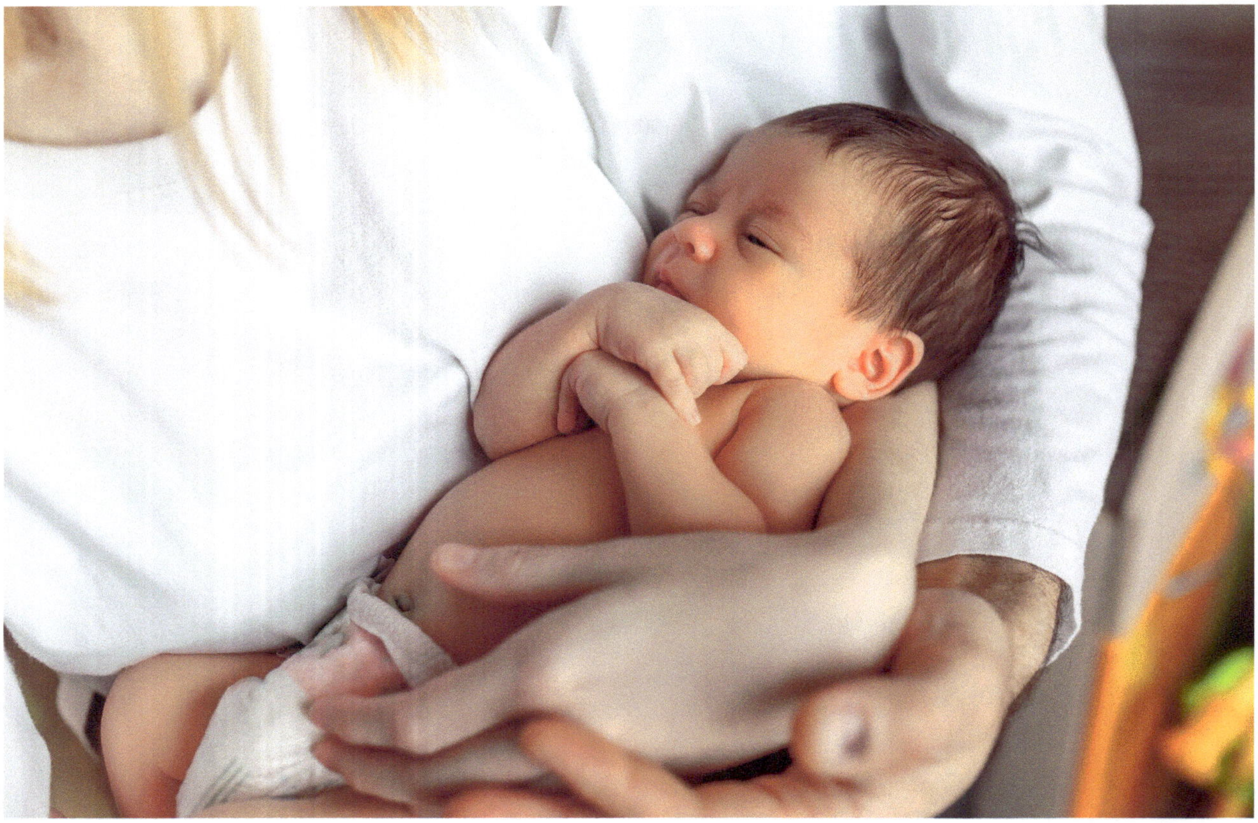

[40] Costello A., Peterson S.S. "Birth in a time of antibiotic-resistant bacteria", *World Health Organization*, 2016.

2.8 Antibiotics and prescriptive appropriateness: three possible interventions to guide doctors

Improving prescriptive appropriateness, especially when it comes to antibiotics and their frequent misuse, can also mean focusing on behavioural aspects that can influence the therapeutic choices of clinicians, especially in outpatient clinics and doctors' surgeries. A recent study verified a number of strategies in order to disincentivise GPs from prescribing antibiotics for the treatment of acute respiratory infections (ARI), revealing how often clinical decisions are influenced by social pressure and pressure from patients (or their parents)[41].

As confirmed by the data of the Italian Medicines Report of the monitoring centre on the use of medicines in Italy, inappropriate use of antibiotics occurs most frequently in the adult population with ARI; indeed, they constitute around 75% of medical interventions in the winter season and 25% of the overall burden of work at GP surgeries. Antibiotics are rarely indicated for the treatment of these diseases, even though they are widely prescribed.

At a national level, 41% of patients with a diagnoses of viral disease of the upper respiratory tract (influenza, colds, acute laryngotracheitis) receive a prescription for antibiotics, even though they are completely useless in the absence of responsible and susceptible bacteria. Moreover, in addition to this inappropriate overprescription, there is also improper use of certain types of antibiotics for disease for which they are absolutely not generally indicated. This is the case with macrolides, fluoroquinolones and cephalosporins, which are wrongly prescribed in one in three cases for treatment of pharyngitis or acute tonsillitis; or injective cephalosporins and fluoroquinolones used for the treatment of acute bronchitis in the absence of asthma or chronic obstructive pulmonary disease (COPD). In Italy, as in the rest of the world, with regard to the clearly very significant cultural phenomenon of erroneous prescription, cases of improper use of antibiotics for infections of the upper respiratory tract are mostly recorded in the south and, in general, in the female population and individuals of advanced age.

The situation in the United States is no different; the number of prescriptions of antibiotics at doctors' and dentists' surgeries, paediatric and outpatient clinics exceeds 250 million, most of which are for the treatment of ARI.

To investigate this phenomenon and possibly to adopt measures to reduce excessive prescription, a randomized trial conducted by a team of researchers from Los Angeles and Boston involved 248 doctors in 47 outpatient clinics for 18 months for the purpose of

[41] Meeker D., Linder J.A., Fox C.R. et al. "Effect of behavioral interventions of inappropriate antibiotic prescribing among primary care practices", *JAMA* 2016;315:562-570.

evaluating three different approaches that might have had potential impact on the treatment choices of the sample patients.

All the interventions made use of an online management system of electronic prescriptions for patients; it was possible to interact directly with the doctor through messages and pop-up dialogue windows or through incoming emails at the time of the prescription. More specifically, with the first intervention, alternative treatments were suggested instead of antibiotics, specifying that these medicines were not appropriate for indicated diagnoses of ARI. The second intervention required clinics to provide a written reason in their own words that justified the prescription of an antibiotic treatment for acute infection of the respiratory tract, with any lack of justification tracked in the system. The third system provided a kind of "classification" based on how many prescriptions for antibiotics were issued by each doctor and continuous comparison with the top performers, that is, those with the lowest number of inappropriate prescriptions.

At the end of the trial period, the results were encouraging for all three methods of discouraging unnecessary prescriptions of antibiotics for the treatment of acute infections of the respiratory tract, with an average percentage decrease in prescriptions of around 5% for each intervention. The two systems of persuasion that envisaged a more "social" type of involvement of the doctor, through, for example, providing written justification and a comparison between colleagues in the prescription of antibiotics, effectively prompted more participants in the trial to prescribe antibiotics more cautiously. The rate of return visits by patients who had not been prescribed antibiotics for the persistence of bacterial infections was also shown to be low.

The added value of this study lies in the simplicity of the proposed interventions, aimed at the precise moment of prescription by clinics and calibrated to rely on the behavioural effect and on the possible impact on the doctor's "image" in the case of inappropriate antibiotic prescription.

The use of the information technology with the electronic prescription also makes the application of these measures very easy and quite cheap, with significant advantages in terms of collective health.

In an editorial commenting on the study, the hope was expressed that this method can also be used to keep better track of prescriptions for antibiotics issued by clinics and to disseminate programmes to manage dispensing of antibiotics, similar to those applied in hospitals[42].

[42] Gerber J.S. "Improving outpatient antibiotic prescribing. Another nudge in the right direction", *JAMA* 2016;315(6):558-559; see also note 41.

2.9 Combatting antimicrobial resistance at the global level. Regulatory initiatives in Europe and in the United States

The "personalised" or "precision" model of medicine that promises to revolutionise the approach to disease and treatment requires the flow and sharing of data and knowledge from different but necessarily associated fields such as new technologies and nanotechnologies, genetics and pharmacology.

The greater the capacity of the system overall to share this knowledge in the early stages of the development of a new medicine (or device), the greater the probability that the time and cost of research can be optimised, reducing the still high failure rate.

The FDA is moving in this direction in the very topical and strategic field of the development of antimicrobial medicines, in which the information from tests of susceptibility to a medicine are particularly valuable in the light of the growing resistance of certain microorganisms to a large number of antimicrobials, even including some introduced recently.

The US agency decided to encourage the developers of antimicrobials and the manufacturers of devices to test antimicrobial susceptibility (AST) to discuss opportunities for coordinated development of their respective products. The discussion – the FDA suggested – should take place at an early stage in the development process. To this end, the US agency drew up a guide, "Coordinated Development of Antimicrobial Drugs and Antimicrobial Susceptibility Test Devices", the first draft of which remained open for public consultation until 21 November 2016[43].

The guide, which contains non-binding recommendations, describes the interactions between the sponsors of an antimicrobial medicine and the manufacturers of AST devices for the coordinated development of the respective products; it also aims to explain the FDA's position with regard to the presentation of separate applications to the Centre for Drug Evaluation (CDER) and the Center for Devices and Radiological Health (CDRH) when authorisation is required for an AST device at the same time or immediately after the approval of an antimicrobial medicine. Finally, the guide seeks to clarify that the review of a new pharmaceutical product and AST devices will remain independent, and that the coordinated development will not influence the expiry dates for the review of each product laid down by the Prescription Drug User Fee Act (PDUFA) and by the Medical Device User Fee Act (MDUFA), respectively.

[43] https://www.fda.gov/downloads/MedicalDevices/DeviceRegulationandGuidance/GuidanceDocuments/UCM521421.pdf?source=govdelivery&utm_medium=email&utm_source=govdelivery.

Antimicrobial susceptibility tests – writes the FDA in the guide – are an important component in supporting the development of new antimicrobial medicines and the subsequent use of these molecules in clinical practice. As well as providing valuable information for the clinical use of antimicrobials, these tests used in epidemiological studies can identify the emergence of resistance to the medicine and monitor the global changes of the population in antimicrobial susceptibility.

The development of antimicrobials and AST devices that test the susceptibility *in vitro* of bacterial pathogens isolated from clinical samples targeting has traditionally been carried out independently – writes the FDA – and often the development of an AST device was begun after the approval of the medicines. Coordinated development would reduce the time between the approval of a new antimicrobial and an AST device that tests *in vitro* the susceptibility of the pathogenic agents to that given molecule. Coordinated development also offers potential benefits, both for the sponsor of the medicine and for the device manufacturer during the respective development processes. Whoever develops the medicine can draw benefit from access to the technology of the device, which may prove useful in the course of clinical trials. The manufacturers of AST devices can, in turn, draw benefit from access to clinical samples obtained during the development of the medicine, which can prove valuable in validating the device. Molecular devices and those that detect antimicrobial resistance through the identification of microbial resistance markers can especially benefit from these advantages.

The nature of these interactions – concludes the FDA – can take many forms and does not have to be limited to a single manufacturer of devices. Making a medicine available to more than one manufacturer of devices during their development can increase their access to clinical laboratories at the time of the approval of the medicine or immediately after.

Another front on which to take action is that of international collaboration between the regulators of the various countries in order to define common standards starting from the clinical trial phase. Aligning the data prerequisites required for clinical trials by regulators throughout the world could contribute to stimulating the development of new antibiotics in order to combat antimicrobial resistance and protect global public health. This is one of the conclusions agreed by the EMA, the Japanese Agency PMDA (Japanese Pharmaceuticals and Medical Devices Agency) and the FDA from a meeting held in London in 2015.

The three agencies agreed on the need to apply certain flexibility to the prerequisites for clinical development programmes of antibacterial agents, especially when the treatment options for patients are limited due to antimicrobial resistance. In light of this, it emerged that it may be appropriate to accept shorter clinical development programmes for new antibiotics able to tackle an unsatisfied need regarding antimicrobial resistance.

In order to better understand the common aspects and the differences between the three regulatory systems in their prerequisites regarding clinical data, attention was focused on approaches to designing clinical trials, including the choice of endpoints and post-authorisation monitoring activities, for antibacterial medicines. Areas for greater collaboration and coordination of efforts to encourage the development of safe and effective antibacterial treatments were also identified.

However, regulatory activities are only one element in a wider and multifaceted response required to encourage and accelerate the development of new antibacterial medicines able to meet the needs of patients.

There has been an upsurge in research worthy of increasing interest in recent years as a result of recent advances in knowledge about the human microbiome, regarding understanding of the connections between the microbiome and infections (among others) with the possibility of developing innovative tools in the fight against antibiotic resistance.

With this aim, the Centers for the Control and Prevention of Diseases (CDC) financed 34 innovative projects for more than US$14 million to investigate new approaches in combatting resistance to antibiotics and, in particular, the way in which microorganisms present naturally in the human body (microbiome) can be used to predict and prevent infections caused by organisms resistant to medicines[44].

This is further support for the Antibiotic Resistance Solutions Initiative of the CDC[45], which aims to implement the monitoring, prevention and management activities of antibiotics outlined in the National Action Plan for Combating Antibiotic-Resistant Bacteria[38].

"Understanding the role that the microbiome plays in infections that are resistant to antibiotics is necessary to protect public health," said the CDC's director, Tom Frieden. "We think that this is the key to innovative approaches able to combat resistance to antibiotics, protect patients and improve the use of antibiotics."

The human microbiome is a vast community of microbes present in nature and in our bodies. Bacteria and other microbes live on our skin, in our intestines, in our mouths and in the respiratory and urinary tracts. A healthy microbiome also helps protect the organism from infections.

The enteric nervous system possesses between 200 and 600 million neurons, a higher number than the entire spinal cord; controlling the intestine requires more intelligence than that required for the rest of the body. And how could it be otherwise? The internal surface of the digestive system is a hundred times larger than the skin area and

[44] https://www.cdc.gov/drugresistance/solutions-initiative/microbiome-innovations.html.
[45] https://www.cdc.gov/drugresistance/solutions-initiative/index.html.

hosts the a boundless family of commensal organisms: 100 trillion made up of 40,000 different species of bacteria, viruses and fungi, and 100 times more genes than the human genome. Eighty percent of our immune system, for example, lies in the intestine, which, like a silent outpost, guards the borders with the external environment and constantly communicates with the internal environment to the point of actually controlling our strategies and our innermost thoughts.

According to this theory, every one of us could therefore belong to a complex mixed species of which only 10% is made up of *Homo sapiens* and the rest of subgroups of Bacteroides, Prevotellae, Ruminococci and many other microorganisms that are yet to be defined in detail but that started to colonise us millions of years ago and are able to modify the development and functioning of our entire body, including the brain. Even in mice, by appropriately changing the intestinal flora (sic!) with anti- and pro-biotics, anxiety levels and motor activity can be changed, that is, the amount of things to be done and the fear that they can evoke. The results from the last three years have lifted the veil on an interesting and curious aspect of the co-evolution of species far back in history. For example, Archaebacteria, which we still host, are able to reproduce and mutate every 20–180 minutes, continuously checking the changes in the environmental conditions. So while the organism that hosts them, the human body, is subject to mutations and evolutionary selections on a scale of at least centuries, our intestines can change the hosted population in a few days. Some diets are immediately followed by a change of intestinal microorganisms and the expression of at least a couple of hundred thousand genes can be modified in a few hours.

If that is hard to believe, we should realise that the signals produced in this way are consciously perceived only in a minority of cases, more precisely only when a consequent motor function is required (feeding or defecating); there is no apparent trace of emotional or behavioural activation of signals that influence memory.

We should respect our gastrointestinal system more and not treat it just as a container that metabolises and eliminates. We are all aware of the hedonistic effect of food (taste and satiation) and the aversion that comes from the irritation of the intestinal mucosae to the point that, after food poisoning, we can no longer eat the food that caused it. We describe this experience, often mistakenly, as a food allergy when, in fact, it has nothing to do with an allergic phenomenon but rather with a sophisticated evolutionary mechanism of learning by association. It is logical to suppose that the first evolutionary signal correlated with food must have been linked to survival. Ingesting food that produces a health benefit for the organism is a behaviour that should be remembered and repeated, whereas food that can potentially cause nausea, intestinal pain or even vomiting must be avoided. We are what we eat or don't eat also applies to our immune defence and our resistance to microorganisms; for this reason,

it is worth "obeying the stomach" every now and again, which has more intelligence than it might seem and could take us much further than we can currently imagine[46].
Antibiotics are lifesaving medicines but they can also harm the microbiome by changing the balance between "good" and "bad" bacteria. "The effects of antibiotics on the microbiome are like a flame in a forest," writes the CDC. Good and bad bacteria, although living in balance, can rapidly be swept away by antibiotics. Resistant bacteria can take advantage of this destruction and multiply, increasing the risk of infection and the spread of resistant bacteria to other individuals.
Patients with microbiomes altered by antibiotics are vulnerable to infections from germs that are "difficult to defeat", such as methicillin-resistant *Staphylococcus aureus*, Enterobacteria resistant to carbapenem (CRE) and *Clostridium difficilis*. These patients can therefore "host" bacteria resistant to medicines that can easily spread to others, especially those with an altered microbiome.
For the most part, financing awarded to US universities rewards studies that investigate the link between antibiotics, the microbiome and the consequences of the widespread use of antibiotics. The research projects will develop in three directions:

- How antibiotics alter a healthy microbiome: in order to determine how early exposure to antibiotics in the course of a life influences the development of the microbiome and to identify new strategies to protect and restore it.

- How an altered microbiome puts health at risk: in order to develop indicators able to prevent the risks to patients who take specific antibiotics, to determine whether these indicators enhance the risk of spreading an infection or of being infected by bacteria resistant to medicines, to develop and test the measurements of the microbiome in order to monitor the risk of a patient and evaluate the effectiveness of greater control of infections in protecting a person's microbiome.

- How the management of an antibiotic can be improved in order to better protect the microbiome: by adapting the strategies of responsible antibiotic management to a patient's individual microbiome and by adapting antibiotic management to meet the needs of different healthcare contexts (for example, hospitals, treatment homes, doctor's surgeries)[47].

[46] Amended by Pani L., Corbellini G. *Imperfezioni umane. Cervello e dissonanze evolutive: malattie e salute tra biologia e cultura* (*Human imperfections. Brain and evolutionary dissonance: diseases straddling biology and culture*), pages 83-86, Rubettino Editore, 2015, Catanzaro.
[47] See note 43; http://www.ema.europa.eu/docs/en_GB/document_library/Other/2016/09/WC500212649.pdf; https://www.cdc.gov/media/releases/2016/p1006-cdc-antibiotic-resistance-research.html.

3. Managing the change: the Government and planning pharmaceutical expenditure

3.1 The "sofosbuvir case". Transparency and responsibility in the "positioning" of innovative medicines

On the matter of sustainable innovation[48], news of the introduction of the first innovative treatment for the hepatitis C virus was widely covered, becoming known as the "sofosbuvir case", an "epoch-making" step in global pharmaceutics that influenced and still influences the agendas and policies of international governments.

We would now like to add a further detail to the story of a medicine that constituted a kind of point of no return, an unequalled precedent for having raised discussion among health systems around the world that grappled with the delicate assessment of how to assign an appropriate price to a treatment that promised to eradicate a serious disease, in compliance with the principle of equal access to treatments and the sustainability of public finances.

This is an indisputably common principle underlying a fundamental question: how to reconcile the inviolable right to health with the assignment of a "right price", able to reward innovation and, at the same time, safeguard the equilibrium of welfare systems?

While we were asking ourselves as early as 2014 – and not just us – on what basis the manufacturer Gilead Sciences had decided the launch price of Sovaldi – the trade name of sofosbuvir – in the United States the chairman of the Senate Finance Commission, Ron Widen, and commissioner Chuck Grassley launched, at the same time and for the same reasons, instigated a formal fact-finding investigation into the pharmaceutical multinational. After a year and a half and an inquiry that analysed more than 20,000 pages of documents provided mainly by Gilead itself in less than 60 days from request, after dozens of interviews of health experts and a vast volume of data from the Medicaid public healthcare programme in 50 states and the district of Washington, DC, the two senators certainly did not use half measures in their conclusions, proclaiming that the company had calculated the initial "positioning" price of its medicine in pursuit of the sole objective of maximising the profit, irrespective of the consequences for people and health systems, as we had suspected in our editorial of July 2014 under the unequivocal title: "From the ethics of profit to the profit of ethics".

"In the correspondence, reports of meetings or presentations," Senators Wyden and Grassley stated during a press conference[49] on the results of the inquiry, "it emerged that, in defining the price of the medicine, basic financial questions, the costs for research and development or even the multibillion acquisition of Pharmasset, the company that had first developed the

[48] Pani L. *L'Innovazione Sostenibile (Sustainable Innovation)*, p. 32 ff. EDRA, 2016, Milan.
[49] https://www.youtube.com/watch?v=rxd_PTFoouo&noredirect=1.

medicine, were not considered. Gilead knew that, with a launch price of US$ 84,000 for 12 weeks' treatment, the medicine would have been out of the reach of millions of people around the world and would certainly have caused problems for the Medicare and Medicaid healthcare programmes in the United States, but it went ahead anyway.
We believe that, if Gilead's approach to deciding the price of Sovaldi is representative of the future strategy for the launch on the market of other potential blockbuster medicines, this would lead to charges of dozens of billions of euros for the treatment of a limited number of patients." In this regard, Senator Wyden stated: "America needs treatments for cancer, Alzheimer's, diabetes and HIV. If these treatments are inaccessible and out of the reach of millions of people who need them, Congress will be falling short in its responsibility to the American people."
Will this also be the scenario for our National Health Service?
We can circle around this as long as we want, but it seems that the entire debate can fundamentally be summed up in two key words: transparency and responsibility. Two words that, to our way of thinking, are crucial in the governance of the policies on medicines. Making a medicine available, for the first time in decades, with such a favourable risk/benefit profile and with such limited adverse effects compared with the treatments previously available[50], and with complete absence of competition, is a bench test for the sense of transparency and responsibility of those who wish to draw a fair profit from it. Fair, certainly, but not colossal. In the United States, Sovaldi remained on the market for nearly a year without competition. In Italy, we did better and negotiated a much lower reimbursement price than the other G8 countries – and probably many others. Within a few months, competition arrived on the market. In the United States, this enabled the company to keep the price very high, notwithstanding the attempts by healthcare programmes and the insurance companies to negotiate discounts or price agreements for high volumes of treatments. In 2014 alone, the federal healthcare coverage programme Medicaid had to spend US$1.3 billion before they could receive the first discounts on the product, managing to guarantee treatment with Sovaldi for less than 2.4% of the 700,000 or so patients with hepatitis C (compared with at least 5 million people who tested positive for the virus). Even though Gilead applied a series of progressive discounts in 2015, prompted by the availability of new treatments for HCV from its competitors, which ousted Sovaldi and Harvoni from the list of medicines of first choice included in insurance policies, the company's revenues continued to reach numbers with nine zeros. In this regard, it is worth remembering that Gilead had a turnover of more

[50] Curry P.M., O'Leary J.G., et al. per ASTRAL-4 Investigators. "Sofosbuvir and Velpatasvir for HCV in Patients with Decompensated Cirrhosis", *N Engl J Med* 2015;373:2618-2628.

than US$ 12 billion in 2014, mostly from anti-HCV medicines, around US$19 billion in 2015 and almost US$30 billion in 2016. None of the financial analysts, probably not even within the company, had forecast these numbers.

Considerations on what would have been a fair cost for the medicine three years after its introduction on the market are not worth commenting upon because it is clear to anyone who understands the so-called drug market take over that there is a period of introduction, a peak period, a plateau and a period of descent. It is obviously not possible now to say that, by imposing unacceptable conditions on the company at that stage in order to treat, as a populist measure, all the individuals who tested positive for HCV (a clinical concept very different from suffering from hepatitis C and its complications), the disease would have been eradicated in three years (sic!), because all those who really needed the medicine would have died in the meantime. The publishers of the *New England Journal of Medicine*[51], citing the results of the aforementioned study that demonstrate the effectiveness and simplicity of a new treatment in association with sofosbuvir, expressed a self-evident and basic truth: no patient will ever be cured if they cannot take a lifesaving medicine that costs too much. This is equivalent to confirming the question the undersigned has raised publicly several times on this matter during the period of the general management of the Italian Medicines Agency: what benefit can ever be offered and what real value can ever be had from an innovative treatment if it literally remains out of the reach of the sick or the healthcare systems? None.

Some questions of a political, socio-economic but also moral nature emerge from the conclusion of the investigation of the American Senate Finance Commission. At this point, after the example of sofosbuvir, we feel it our duty to ask whether, for every promising new treatment that may come on the market, we will have sufficient knowledge of its effective costs, the pool of patients who can benefit from it and confirmation of its greater efficacy. What does "value" really mean in defining the price of a medicine and what instruments can be deployed to sustain the utmost transparency in the negotiation processes, at the same time ensuring the necessary incentives for those who develop such effective new treatments?

The American senators were especially concerned about population of low earners and the sustainability of healthcare programmes. This is not the case in Italy, unique in the world for its universal and community-based National Health Service, for the time being.

We join the call for greater transparency with conviction because an increasing number of innovative medicines will soon be available for the treatment of cancers and dementia – just

[51] Ward J.W., Mermin J.H. "Simple, effective, but out of reach? Public health implications of HCV drugs", *N Engl J Med* 2015;373:2678-2680.

to mention a few – and having clarity of information about the costs sustained in their development in order to calculate fair profit will become fundamental.

To the data from the American Senate investigation, we add further information contained in a report[52] published by the Americans for Tax Fairness (ATF) and picked up by *Bloomberg*[53], according to which Gilead allegedly made use of accountancy expedients to transfer earnings of billions to off-shore tax paradises.

"Since the pharmaceutical multinational introduced the medicine at 1000 dollars a day for hepatitis C, its profit margin soared dramatically while its tax rate dropped by 40%," the report's authors claimed. By transferring some of its intellectual property to Ireland, Gilead allegedly adopted a strategy deployed by other American companies (see recent similar cases involving Apple) which enabled it to reduce US taxes by US$10 billion from 2013.

Two thirds of the sales of Sovaldi were made in the United States but Gilead paid taxes on only around 37% of its profits on national territory, assigning the remaining percentage to locations with no or reduced taxation.

The company's profit margin – the report continued – increased fivefold from 2013 and last year reached US$21.7 billion, according to the documents published by the company. In the same period, Gilead's tax rate globally fell from 27.3% to 16.4%. Even though the mandatory tax rate on companies in the United States is 35%, most companies pay much less and Gilead does not disclose its actual tax rate in the United States.

The report describes as "particularly irritating" the evasion of US federal taxes, because federal research grants (NIH and the Department of Veterans' Affairs) contributed to making the development of Sovaldi possible. "US taxpayers paid Gilead 5 billion dollars a year for the treatment of thousands of patients suffering from hepatitis C through Medicare and Medicaid," the authors continued, criticising the aggressive pricing policy practiced by the company. When it was introduced in 2013, the 12-week treatment cycle had a list price of US$84,000, before the discounts and lower prices negotiated with the insurance companies – the report recalls – while Harvoni, a combined treatment that associated sofosbuvir with ledipasvir, also owned by Gilead, debuted a year later at US$1125 a tablet, or US$94,500 for a complete treatment. Yet "various research groups estimated the cost of production of a complete treatment of between 68 and 1400 dollars". From the experience with the sofosbuvir case, the Italian Medicines Agency, thanks to its commissions (Scientific Technical Commission and Prices and Reimbursements Committee) and the aid of scientific societies and patients' associations, learned important lessons: on the one hand, it was an opportunity

[52] https://americansfortaxfairness.org/new-report-gilead-sciences-price-gouger-tax-dodger/.

[53] Kocieniewski D. "Gilead seen cutting taxes by $10 billion as pricey drug took off", *Bloomberg* 2016.

to outline and apply new paradigms for deciding an adequate price, based on the degree of innovation of this new molecule and the health effect produced; on the other hand, a price negotiation strategy was pursued for Sovaldi, taking into consideration all the other valid therapeutic alternatives that would soon be available. This is perhaps why the Italian Medicines Agency was the first European Agency to deem the manufacturer's initial economic request excessive and inadmissible from the ethical and financial point of view. It must be remembered that, to enable access to the treatment, additional funds were necessary, which the Health Minister requested and promptly defended with far-sightedness, and the foundations were laid for an ambitious public health plan to attempt to eradicate hepatitis C in Italy in the very near future; realistically, however, as stated by the WHO, this could take several decades[54]. This plan ought reasonably to be developed in the coming years, a period in which it can be hoped that better definition of the actual number of eligible patients may be possible; screening would enable the virus to be detected before the development of organ-damaging disease and, above all, the effects of all the treatments available in actual clinical practice could be verified thanks to the monitoring registers. From the perspective of increasing transparency, an initiative was launched in December 2015 to provide information weekly on the institutional website of the Italian Medicines Agency, regarding the state of progress of treatments for HCV in Italy. By 13 November 2017, more than 100,000 patients (based on the various eligibility criteria)[55] had begun the first treatment, among all the therapies available. As the Italian Medicines Agency has made clear many times, there can be no innovation and fair access to medicines without ensuring that the costs are sustainable. The price policies of the companies cannot be guided only by the logic of profit, which does not take into account the long-term ethical and strategic repercussions, because this would be to the detriment not only of patients but also the research that gives rise both to the health benefits for the community and "healthy" profits for businesses. In the face of evidence of this kind, if confirmed, it would be legitimate to suspect that Gilead is not only a pharmaceutical but rather a financial company and that its strategies to continue to maximise profits are seriously obfuscating not only its image but also its global commercial value. All this would produce much greater economic damage than expected, something that its renewed management would do well to take account. In confirmation of this forecast, the value of Gilead quoted on Wall Street, notwithstanding the therapeutic and economic financial success of its anti-HCV products, indicated a loss of around 50% from June 2015 to June 2017.

[54] http://www.quotidianosanita.it/allegati/allegato2649130.pdf.

[55] http://www.aifa.gov.it/sites/default/files/Aggiornamento_dati_Registri_AIFA_DAAs_13-11-2017.pdf.

3.2 Innovative strategies for the sustainability of pharmaceutical expenditure: the example of the Italian Medicines Agency in Europe and in the international press

As never before, the price of medicines has become a dominant issue in public opinion, in political debates, and on the agendas of traditional and social media. If the new direct-action antivirals against the hepatitis virus have blazed the trail, traumatically testing the capacity for adaptation and response of the health systems, other new high-cost molecules, also intended to modify the therapeutic strategies for highly prevalent diseases, are landing on the market with an impact that is difficult to assess according to the paradigms that have been established in recent decades. Increasingly, international analysts look to the Italian model with attention and interest and the strategies that our country is deploying to tackle the new scenarios.

The primary difference in Italy is a National Health Service that, to date, covers more than 75% of the global expenditure for the acquisition of medicines, guaranteeing its citizens a range of treatments that include low-cost equivalent medicines and monoclonal antibodies or gene therapies. This is a level of performance that only an entirely public system like ours is able to achieve, succeeding where other countries, where healthcare is entrusted to private or mixed system, have often failed.

Obamacare – Giuseppe Remuzzi[56] observed at the presentation of the book *Sustainable Innovation* on 14 June 2016 – was a praiseworthy and courageous attempt but, notwithstanding the enormous investment, it did not achieve the hoped-for effects "because a system so rooted in strong and consolidated interests as the American model is difficult to break up". On the contrary, Italy, which succeeded in retaining the universal and community-based nature of its National Health Service, faces an arduous but possible task: rationalising and modernising the system to ensure its survival and efficiency.

Personally, I have always believed that this challenge can only be met with reform at the national level, without delegation to the regions but with their participation and collaboration in order to make the best practices of the virtuous a common factor, immediately placing under a commissioner those that have consistently shown, for the last 5 years for example, that they are not able to manage the enormous resources of the National Healthcare Fund that are allocated to them.

Another Italian prerogative concerns the regulatory model. The Italian Medicines Agency, unlike other agencies that do not have responsibility for setting the prices of medicines,

[56] http://www.marionegri.it/it_IT/home/istituto/chi_siamo/biografie/giuseppe_remuzzi.

manages both the risk/benefit assessments and the cost/benefit assessments, with the advantage of being able to harmonise authorisation activities with release on the market, price negotiations and reimbursement decisions.

At the European level, where the aim is "rapid access to innovative medicines at a sustainable price", there is an increasing need to make a connection between authorisation for release on the market, scientific evaluations and Health Technology Assessment (HTA) and decisions on prices. This is what Italy has already been doing for several years with instruments such as parallel HTA and scientific advice, conditional authorisation, reimbursement models based on results (payment by results) and monitoring registers. It is precisely this unique feature that has enabled, among other things, negotiations for very costly medicines between 2011 and 2016, such as anti-cancer and direct-action antivirals against hepatitis C, at significantly lower prices than the European average, ensuring the efficiency and speed of the entire regulatory process.

Confirmation of this was provided by a report by Karl Broich[57], chairman of the German Federal Institute for Drugs and Medical Devices (Bfarm) at a meeting of the HMA (Heads of Medicines Agencies) held in June 2016 in Rotterdam during the Dutch Presidency of the EU. In his speech ("Gateway between the approval, reimbursement and affordability role of regulators"), Broich, citing the latest report by IMS Health[58], compared the average times of access to medicines in the United States, European Union Five – EU5 (French, Germany, Italy, Spain and the United Kingdom) and the rest of Europe.

According to the IMS Health data for 2014, Italy was in eighteenth place (out of 22 countries) for the average times of access to a medicine on the market after regulatory approval (14.5 months). Only Greece, Romania, Russia and Spain recorded longer times. This is a half-truth that, in recent years, has been paraded to the delight of the average industrialist or trade association, both directly and indirectly through scientific societies (sic!) or federations representing this or that group. On the contrary, when the average time for marketing authorisation and the final decision on prices and reimbursement are considered, Italy has the lowest average time among the EU5 (0.7 months compared with 2.3 in Spain, 4.6 in France, 11 in the United Kingdom and 12.7 in Germany) and, thanks to this performance, is in second place, after the United Kingdom, for the average total time between authorisation of a medicine and its availability, entirely at the expense of the Health Service, on national territory

[57] Broich is one of the authors, together with EMA's Executive Director, Guido Rasi, Senior Medical Office Hans-Georg Eichler, Executive Director of the *Dutch Medicines Evaluation Board, Hugo Hurts, of a recent article* ("Drug regulation and pricing – can regulators influence affordability?") published in the *New England Journal of Medicine* on access to medicines and the role of the regulators.

[58] https://www.imshealth.com/files/web/Global/Services/P&MA_2015.pdf.

following the negotiation procedure and the definition of the reimbursement regime. As always, intellectual honesty and the real absence of conflicts of interest would have helped give citizens more factual information that would have reinforced the sense of trust in those institutions doing their duty.

These are data that refute the lie on the common assumption according to which Italy has an excessively long authorisation and negotiation procedure that acts as a barrier to prompt access to new medicines for patients. On the contrary, the data confirm the wisdom of entrusting the entire decision-making process to a single authority.

Figura 1 - Average times (months) from regulatory approval to the release on the market – products released in 2014.

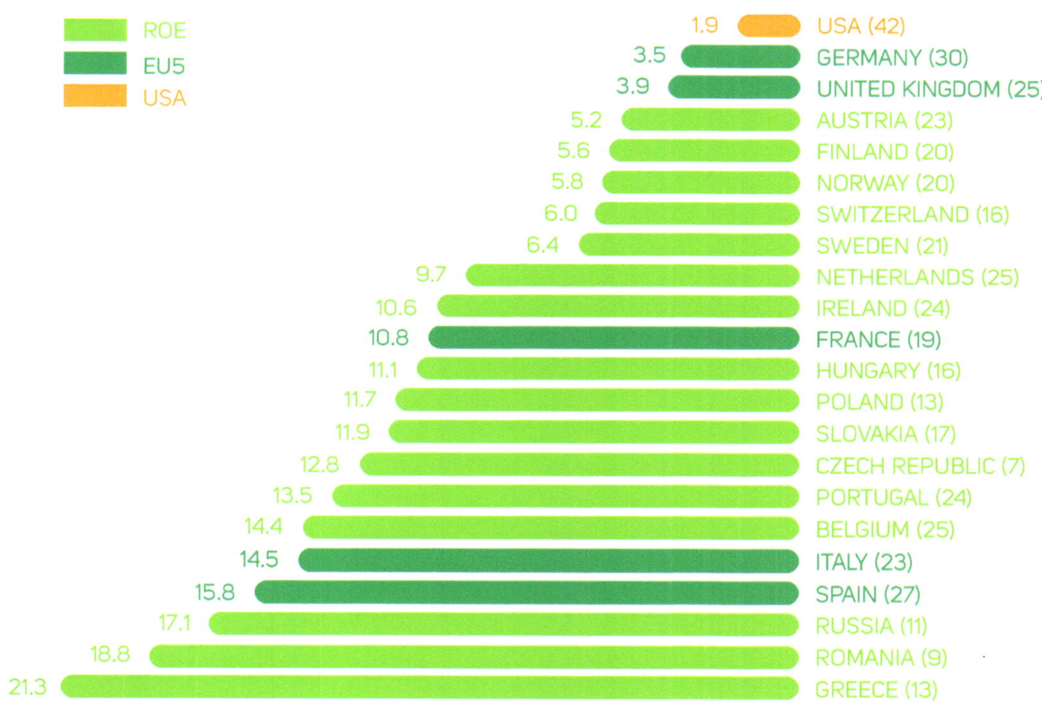

Figura 2 - Average times (months) from regulatory approval to release on the market and from release on the market to approval by the National Pharma in 2014.

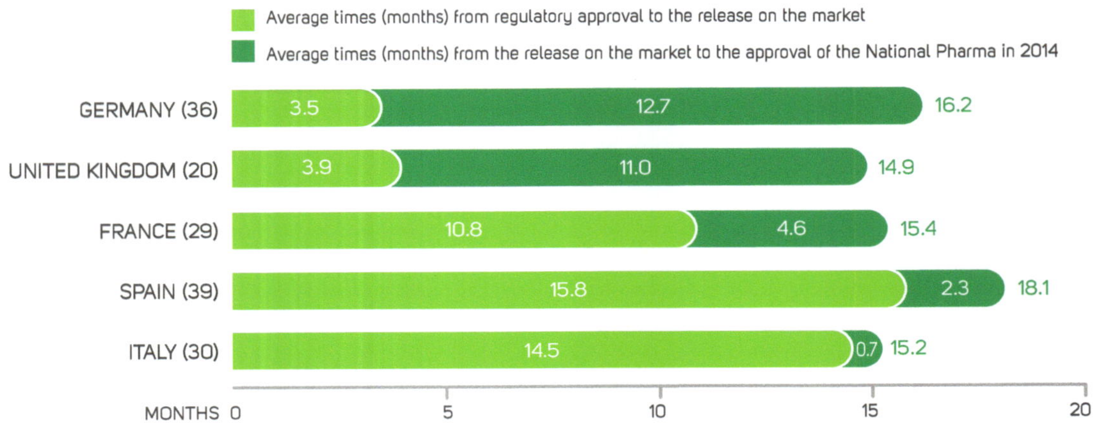

Recently, moreover, the conditional reimbursement models used by the Italian Medicines Agency in the negotiation procedures for new medicines have attracted admiration even in the United States by *Bloomberg*'s pharmaceutical economic analysis services[59].
An idea launched some time ago by the Italian Medicines Agency and shared by the authors of these articles is that the "Made in Italy" concept should be extended beyond the traditional stereotypes of success (fashion and cars) to also include, necessarily, innovative leadership strategies for the control of pharmaceutical expenditure deployed during the five-year period from 2011 to 2016.
"The Italian Medicines Agency," wrote Makiko Kitamura and Johannes Koch, "has concluded agreements with the pharmaceutical companies under which the payment of medicines takes place on the basis of how much and how the way a patient responds to the treatment and, in cases where the medicine produces no effect, the company repays the entire cost. Italy has initialled an increasing number of agreements of this type, since the number of medicines that receive approval after an intermediate phase trial conducted on at least 100 patients are boosting, rather than wait for the final phase involving thousands of people."

[59] Kitamura M., Koch J. "When cancer treatments fail Italy wants money back", *Bloomberg* 2016.

The Italian Medicines Agency is very probably the first regulatory body in the world to have provided advanced application of various models of conditional reimbursement. These agreements (MEAs – Managed Entry Agreements) were originally divided into two main categories: agreements to share the risk based on outcomes (performance-based risk-sharing schemes such as payment by results, risk sharing and success fees) and agreements of a strictly financial nature (financial-based schemes such as cost sharing and capping).
Vital support for these negotiation models is currently provided by the new monitoring registers adopted by the Agency, truly dynamic databases that assess the use of medicines in clinical practice, gathering the data, in full respect of privacy, on hundreds of thousands of individual treatments at the level of the individual patient.
According to the latest update[60], around 142 monitoring registers have been activated[61] by the Italian Medicines Agency and associated with the various types of negotiation agreements. Specifically, 45 products were subject to monitoring (verification of the prescriptive appropriateness) that involved a performance-based risk-sharing arrangement (PBRSA), that is, 100% refunds in the event of failure of the treatment, 24 products with financial-based arrangements (FBA) and 2 products with a combination of PBRSA and FBA. For 71 products, the aim was only verification of the prescriptive appropriateness.
The global revolution underway in the pharmaceutical world is, in effect, putting traditional pharmaco-economic approaches under great stress everywhere and, more generally, pharmaceutical and healthcare policies. In this context, international observers and stakeholders recognise the peculiarity of the Italian system, which is studied with interest in the United States and in the rest of Europe, where, as the researcher of the London School of Economics, Olivier Wouters, observes, there are no models with the same level of detail and complexity.
In France, where a national register does not exist, Roche launched a pilot programme in 24 hospitals in the last two years to understand the difficulties in monitoring patient and treatment results. The United Kingdom tried out the strategy of result-based prices, but the last contract under this method dates back to 2007, when Johnson & Johnson agreed full reimbursement if its medicine Velcade for blood tumours did not contribute to prolonging the survival of patients[59].
The Italian Medicines Agency established the registers with stunning foresight in 2005 and, in the last five years, they have been transformed and significantly boosted, and

[60] Update of 29 September 2017 http://www.agenziafarmaco.gov.it/content/registri-farmaci-sottoposti-monitoraggio.
[61] Registers Table and active PTs reference http://www.aifa.gov.it/content/lista-aggiornata-dei-registri-e-dei-piani-terapeutici-web-based.

are now considered to be a strategic resource from the regulatory point of view. In order to regulate innovation, an integrated approach is required that can exploit the synergy between the scientific evaluations, the information from the HTA and the pharmacological data in a constantly self-perpetuating cycle.

This is a system that, in addition to enabling granular monitoring, made possible the recovery of more than €200 million for ineffective treatments in 2015, the equivalent of 1% of national pharmaceutical expenditure. The use of agreements for sharing the risk based on results maximises effectiveness, ensures respect for prescriptive appropriateness and, at the same time, enables the sustainability of pharmaceutical expenditure to be safeguarded.

3.3 Prices of medicines in Europe: a European Commission report examining pricing strategies in-depth

High-cost medicines are the most difficult challenge to overcome, both within the European Union and overseas, and, for this reason, analyses are underway – on many fronts – on the most effective policies to keep prices under control, ensuring, at the same times, access for citizens, control of public budgets and support for innovation.
This is the most important objective both for the responsible national authorities and the public payers due to the fact that the price and reimbursement policies of medicines remain the responsibility of the member states of the European Union.
In the European context, the Italian model stands out not only because, as already mentioned, both authorisation and negotiation and the decisions on the reimbursement of medicines are under the responsibility of the same authority, that is, the Italian Medicines Agency, but also because the Italian Agency considers a multiplicity of instruments, some of which are innovative.
As is known, negotiation of prices in Italy takes place in accordance with the following criteria: cost/effectiveness ratio, cost/treatment ratio and cost/per day compared with products of similar effectiveness and safety with the same therapeutic indications; assessment of the economic impact on the National Health Service; market shares; and estimates of patients eligible for the treatment with the new medicine; as well as price and consumption benchmarks in other European countries. These activities are supplemented with data from the OsMed Monitoring Centre and the evaluation of HTA studies and supported by the use of the Italian Medicines Agency monitoring registers and the reimbursement instruments of the Managed Entry Agreements, and by sharing the economic risks with the companies (conditional reimbursement schemes).
However, as pointed out by the Italian Medicines Agency on various occasions, the incoming wave of innovation makes it increasingly urgent to assess the appropriateness and feasibility of a synergic action at the supranational level. For this reason, the initiation of consideration of these issues in the European Union can only be a good omen.
From this perspective, a consortium made up of universities and research institutes in Austria and Luxembourg was commissioned by the European Commission to explore two options: an external reference price (EPR) and a differential price system (DP). The aim of the assessment was to examine the potential arising from the adoption of these two instruments in achieving the objectives mentioned previously: improving access to medicines for patients and, at the same time, generating savings for taxpayers.

Although with different approaches and methods, ERP (also known as setting prices through international benchmarking) is used in 20 European countries of 32 examined as the only or the main price policy, even though the use of pharmaco-economic and HTA assessments for new medicines is increasing.

To apply this system, member states establish a "basket" of comparison with other countries, with prices used as indicators to establish the price of medicines in the internal market and taking numerous factors into consideration.

With regard to the objective of access – the Report's authors[62] observed that ERP has certain limits: it incentivises, for example, market authorisation holders to launch their products first in countries with the highest price levels so that the list prices, where these are highest, can later be used as a reference for setting prices in other countries, to the point of delaying the launch or even not marketing some medicines in countries with lower price levels. The lack of some medicines, seen increasingly often in some European countries in recent years, as well as the convergence on prices, could be partly attributable to the industry's strategic product launches in response to the ERP mechanism.

In any event, ERP has been shown to generates savings for the paying public in certain countries, at least in the short term. Twenty-two of the 32 countries examined reported the use of discounts, rebates or confidential agreements (MEA). These are instruments that enable savings to be generated for the public budgets of countries that use them, while those that use these prices as references do not benefit from the same price reduction. The selection of the panel of countries for comparison can also produce different effects in terms of savings and access. One proposal is to select countries with similar economic contexts, making reference to weighted prices on the basis of the GDP or purchasing power (PPP). Moreover, exchange of information and good practices between member states would be desirable, in particular through the existing instruments, such as the European database of prices of medicines (Euripid)[63].

The DP mechanism, which consists of a policy of governments (or of international institutions) to set the prices of medicines on the basis of the ability to pay and/or the economic situation of the countries, is not applied in the pharmaceutical field in Europe. The literature suggests use on a low scale, typically in countries with low or average income, for specific groups of medicines (vaccines and medicines against HIV/AIDS, tuberculosis and malaria). There are very few examples of collaborative approaches among governments (for example,

[62] Study on enhanced cross-country coordination in the area of pharmaceutical product pricing – Final Report Funded by the Health Programme of the European Union, 2015.

[63] https://euripid.eu.

in Central America) for jointly setting DPs: most often the decision is taken at the central level by agencies or international programmes such as UNICEF. In these cases, the DP was introduced with the aim of ensuring access to medicines that otherwise would not have been provided in those markets. Some prerequisites for the effective use of the DP are the feasibility of competitive production, the need for rapid access to small quantities of medicines and the lack of a market before the introduction of the DP system. This latter premise is also the most likely reason that DP may not be successful in improving access for patients in average income countries, where the markets already exist[64].

Where the DP has been applied, it has been seen more as a criterion for improving access than as an instrument for containing costs. Competition, especially the entry of genetic medicines, was actually shown to be more effective for the second objective. The two limits of DP most often mentioned are the existence of a parallel trade that leads to the "flight" of medicines from countries with lower prices to those where prices are higher, and the widespread use of EPR, which would not incentivise pharmaceutical companies to offer lower prices to countries with low incomes.

The main presupposition for the introduction of a DP system for selected categories of medicines, for example, would be the agreement of member states on the principles and mechanisms of this new collaborative approach. The implementation of a DP system would require the acceptance and commitment to supply costly medicines to low income countries at significantly lower prices. In this way, high-income countries, by sustaining higher prices, would contribute to a greater share of the research and development of the medicines that are unquestionably of global public benefit[65].

Because there has been no experience with DPs in high-income countries, it would be desirable to conduct one or more pilot projects on high-cost medicines, such as orphan medicines or medicines with therapeutic benefits that are expected to be high. The identification of a candidate medicine could take place through early dialogue among regulators, HTA bodies and payers, on the model of other pilot projects such as the "adaptive pathways" (Adaptive Licensing/Pathways – MAAPs) and the MoCA project (mechanism of coordinated access to orphan medicines)[66].

According to the European Commission's Report, EU member states must decide whether to opt for technical improvement of the EPR system that they can implement unilaterally, helping to guarantee the sustainability of the system, or, alternatively, take certain

[64] https://pricingsociety.com/wp-content/uploads/2016/07/Why_Pricing_Strategies_Fail.pdf.
[65] http://www.aei.org/wp-content/uploads/2011/10/20070808_22039HP009Bate_g.pdf.
[66] http://www.eurordis.org/content/moca.

socio-economic characteristics on price matters into consideration, unilaterally or with a collaborative approach, such as a DP system, as a measure for improving access.

The full introduction of a differentiated price system in Europe, although not entirely impossible, would nevertheless require central coordination in order to tackle obstacles currently relevant in legal, technical, organisational and political terms, and would not be the most desirable choice to tackle the challenges involved in fair access to medicines. The report therefore recommends concentrating on improvements to be made to the systems based on the external reference price currently in existence, as a first concrete step.

This study only examined two types of polices (EPR and DP), given that other price determination strategies, including reimbursement strictly tied to price (such as a price based on value, HTA, pharmaco-economic assessments and MEAs) did not come within the range of the inquiry. It would therefore be desirable to carry out additional surveys, without limiting the field of application to these two price policies[66]. This is something that, together with other highly specialised colleagues, we are trying to implement in various parts of the world, but interestingly no longer in Italy where – we hope to be proved wrong – we can expect a regression in the capacity and negotiating conditions in the coming years.

The debate on the definition of a "fair" price for medicines continues but the need to involve other interested parties, in addition to the regulatory authorities and the industry, is increasingly evident. In the future, multi-stakeholder round tables will acquire greater weight, within which the interested parties, primarily the patients, can openly debate without being bound by an institutional mandate. This dialogue could enable alternative solutions to emerge in order to solve this problem, which is rapidly becoming a crucial question worldwide.

3.4 Pharmaceutical research, access to innovation and sustainable price policies. Towards new models of collaboration between stakeholders

On this issue of the price of medicines, a report[67] was recently produced by the Pharma Diplomacy Working Group, made up of representatives from the industry, health systems, HTA organisations, patients' associations and government consultants from Europe and the United States. The Group identified the issue as "the current major source of distrust between the pharmaceutical industry and its stakeholders, although certainly not the only one" and proposed certain considerations, making clear the various points of view.

For health systems, the growing pressure of costs due to the increase in the average prices of medicines is combined with demographic and epidemiological trends and with the processes of reform of the health sector, seriously threatening their sustainability. From the point of view of many patients, concerns regarding accessibility to new medicines are becoming increasingly personal. Especially in countries where citizens contribute to co-financing healthcare, attention to the issue of the price of the new medicines has noticeably increased, not least because, in some cases, insurers are transferring the greater cost of pharmaceutical products to the patients through higher levels of excess and higher co-payments, sometimes in the form of co-insurance policies. In this way, citizens are being forced to pay a greater share than in the past (up to 40–60% in the case of some proprietary medicines).

According to a report by the Kaiser Family Foundation published in September 2015, patients in the United States, for example, have seen their insurance excess increase six times faster than their salaries since 2010. The result is a greater sensitivity among patients about out-of-pocket expenses for medicines and a growing involvement in the discussion on prices.

For its part, the industry argues, and probably not entirely without foundation, that the public rhetoric on prices is also a distraction from the inefficiencies of health systems and limited investments, that the share of expenditure on pharmaceutical products of the total for healthcare is the same today as it was in 1960, and that pharmaceutical innovation, which is producing targeted and highly effective treatments, must be paid for, not only to cover the costs of research and development but, above all, to incentivise investors to sustain future innovation.

These diverging points of view tend to polarise further due to the scarcity of mechanisms able to encourage the various actors to agree on shared solutions. The parties concerned – patients,

[67] Principles for Collaborative, Mutually Acceptable Drug Pricing. Conclusions of the Pharma Diplomacy Dialogue, 2016; https://issuu.com/meteos1/docs/pharmadiplomacy-report-low-res.

taxpayers, pharmaceutical companies and doctors – do not agree on what constitutes "value" for a medicine, on which clinical results can be considered significant, or on the evidence required to justify them. We devoted a long and detailed essay to this subject[68].

The main cause for distrust over prices, however, seems to arise from the lack of transparency in the way companies decide on prices for new medicines. These concerns led to regulations on transparency concerning medicines registered in Massachusetts, California, North Carolina, New York and Pennsylvania, which require pharmaceutical companies to disclose the development costs in order to justify price increases.

Payers have also had to deal with the increase in the prices of proprietary medicines. They have done so by negotiating hard to obtain the maximum discounts, intervening on the criteria and priorities for the prescription of medicines, adopting, as happened in the United States, policies of exclusion, limiting the number of available treatments by therapeutic area and forcing companies to make offers in competition with each other. Some payers are also setting limits on price increases for medicines that will enable treatments to be retained in the formulary (so-called inflation protection) and others are introducing new, onerous conditions for early authorisation. In this way, the initiatives taken by the payers in the United States to deal with price inflation range from entry of a greater number of equivalent or replacement medicines in the formulary to the increasingly extensive use of the HTA, to the role of independent organisations like the Institute for Clinical and Economic Review (ICER) in assessing the cost/effectiveness ratio and the impact on the budget, and in the definition of the price based on value (ICER promises 15–20 reviews of high-impact medicines between 2016 and 2018). In Europe in recent years, the European Council invited the European Commission and national governments to cooperate for the development of "strategies for the management of the expenditure for pharmaceutical products and medical devices, ensuring fair access to effective medicines within sustainable national health systems".

However, acknowledging the need to maintain a balance between attracting innovation and the management of health expenditure, European Health Ministers invited national governments and the European Commission to cooperate more closely on a "life cycle approach" for new innovative medicines. There is also a growing drive to undertake multinational purchase agreements that can be of particular importance in the long term. Belgium and the Netherlands signed an agreement for orphan medicines in April 2015. Bulgaria and Romania say they are ready to follow that example for a potentially wider range of products even if, it must be said, the results are currently rather disappointing.

---

[68] Corbellini G., Pani L. "Prescrivere Valore. Storia e Scienza dei Farmaci che ci fanno vivere più a lungo e meglio" (*Prescribing values. History and science of medicine that make us live longer and better*). EDRA-LSWR, 2017, Milan.

The point of view of patients is also increasingly influential in the debates on price as much in Europe, where an organisation like EURORDIS exists, as in the United State, where the Patient-Centered Value Model Rubric should be mentioned. An active role is also being carved out by doctors through the creation of "medicine assessment instruments" (for example, DrugAbacus[69], developed by Peter Bach of the Memorial Sloan Kettering Cancer Center and colleagues, for the assessment of treatments against cancer), the doctors' associations and the authorities that draw up the guidelines.

The American Society of Clinical Oncology (ASCO) launched a value framework to compare new cancer treatments on the basis of the clinical benefits and toxicity. Alongside a score for "net benefit for health", the purchase costs for the medicines on the list are entered to help doctors and their patients make an informed choice.

The National Comprehensive Cancer Network (NCCN), widely acknowledged in the United States as the standard setter for clinical guidelines in oncology, has become the latest institute to introduce costs in its assessments. In October 2015, the "Affordability of Regimen" was published, a compendium of the costs of medicines that includes, in addition to the prices, the associated costs, including administrative and hospital costs and/or monitoring of the toxicity.

To be fully effective, however, any value framework must also be informed and guided by the systematic inclusion of the perspectives of the patients, who have unique knowledge, perspectives and experience of vital importance, different from that of doctors, researchers, taxpayers and pharmaceutical companies.

Those who invest in pharmaceutics – a very diverse panorama – also have a role in determining the prices of medicines. Indeed, the Pharma Industry is under pressure to satisfy the short-term expectations of those investors who see pharmaceutical shares as a trading opportunity rather than a long-term investment. This drives companies to request the highest possible price at the time of the launch, despite concerns over the reaction of the public and the payers.

After a period of low productivity in research and development, investors seem more optimistic about the future of pharmaceutical innovation but realise that the growing social disquiet about the prices of medicines requires careful monitoring. Some are waiting expectantly, others see the development of prices through more suspicious eyes and hope the companies can convincingly distinguish between breakthrough innovation and incremental innovation. However, even breakthrough innovation, according to some, must have a more reasonable price in order to avoid excessive repercussions in the system.

[69] http://www.drugabacus.org/.

Still others are worried about the long-term consequences. These investors fear that some extreme behaviours on prices introduce a destabilising risk for the pharmaceutical market; they argue that the current price models are not sustainable and see individual developments such as Pooled European Procurement (the only European contract), growing patient activism, the policy debate on the question of the prices of medicines and an increased interest in evidence from the real world, as early signs of more profound changes in the area of prices.

As with all the developments that directly concern health, in this case, the effects of the "revolution" that is underway are also immediately having an impact on citizens; unexpected prospects of cures and improvements in the quality of life raise questions, perhaps for the first time with equal force, such as programmed access to new medicines and, in mixed or mainly private systems, increasing charges from sharing costs that are becoming increasingly unsustainable both for public budgets and for private healthcare programmes.

Fair and prompt access to pharmaceutical innovation, the promotion of research and price policies that are sustainable for health systems are the closely correlated objectives for the near future. To achieve these objectives, all the stakeholders (payers, regulators, patients, researchers, the industry and financial backers) must engage in dialogue in a context of responsibility, reciprocal trust and acknowledgement of roles and expertise.

4. The new frontiers of medicine

4.1 The future of medicine: a pact between "intelligences"

To sufficiently understand what awaits us in the governance of new treatments, we have drawn up some ideas around a series of facts on the new frontiers of medicine or, as we will see, what will remain of biology, pharmaceutics and medicine itself in the coming years.
JAMA, for example, recently explored the potential of artificial intelligence applied in a particular way to the world of health, with a focus on one of its most innovative capacities, that of automatic learning, better known in the literature as deep machine learning.
The term was coined for the first time by Arthur Samuel in 1950, a pioneer in artificial intelligence and the true father of the discipline, defined by him as the "field of study that gives computers the ability to learn (and to carry out a task) without being explicitly programmed to do it".
The expression "artificial intelligence"[70], on the other hand, was used for the first time in the 1950s by the cognitive scientist John McCarthy, who defined it as "the science and design of intelligent machines" and its purpose was not to replicate human intelligence, an aim that for some is utterly unacceptable, but rather to reproduce it or to emulate some of its functions.
Automatic learning, instead, takes place through the creation of systems and algorithms aimed at observing and capturing information directly from data for the synthesis of new knowledge without using a predetermined equation as a model.
Machine learning models are used in numerous applications, such as computational finance, computational biology (detecting tumours, pharmacological identification and DNA sequencing), the production of energy, automatic processing of natural language, image and sound recognition, marketing or for automatic suggestion.
The issue is very topical and debated at the international level. Consider the analysis "Artificial Intelligence & Cognitive Computing Systems in Healthcare" produced by Frost & Sullivan, a US consultancy agency for market analysis and research.
The report reveals that the artificial intelligence market in the health sector produced income of US$633.8 million in 2014 and estimates that this figure will reach US$6662.2 billion in 2021, with a compound annual growth rate of around 40%.
Artificial intelligence systems, which already play an important role in other sectors, are destined to transform the way we think about the diagnosis and treatment of diseases and, by increasing the expertise of qualified doctors, will provide an additional level of decision-making support, able to help reduce oversights and errors in the administration of treatments.

[70] http://www.treccani.it/enciclopedia/intelligenza-artificiale_%28Enciclopedia-della-Scienza-e-della-Tecnica%29/.

The clinical support offered by artificial intelligence systems will reinforce diagnostic imaging processes in the medical field. Moreover, the use of artificial intelligence solutions in the workflow will improve the administration of treatments. Overall, artificial intelligence has the potential to improve treatment outcomes by 30–40%, at the same time reducing the costs by up to 50%.

In the study published in *JAMA*, the authors report some specific experiences of the use of technological instruments linked to automatic learning and show the need for the healthcare world to fully "exploit" the potential of artificial intelligence systems.

The dissemination of mobile devices and the adoption of wearable technologies on a wide scale has given a dimension to machine learning that was entirely unexpected only a few years ago, enabling the loading of large quantities of personal data in (self) learning algorithms: consider the smartphone, no longer as a biometric device but also as a platform from which to initiate tailor-made interventions based on algorithms, continuously optimised to provide personal information in real time.

Among the examples, a specific algorithm has been created based on automatic learning and constructed using decision trees and nested analytical structures that has enabled the number of steps to be reduced (from 29 to 8, to be precise) required for the diagnosis of autistic spectrum disorders (ASD) with a precision of 100% among 612 patients with ASD.

Another example is the possibility that wearable devices can improve treatment for diabetes, registering glycaemia through a small gauge placed on the upper part of the arm. The data are easily sent to the patient's smartphone and then to the GP for checking. In this regard, a study has shown that a glucose sensor linked to an insulin pump can reduce nocturnal hypoglycaemia[71].

Moreover, mobile technology can also extract models and meanings from processing the tracking of daily language and so-called sentiment analysis. For example, a cellular telephone can recognise speech models associated with "thought disorders" by simply listening to the speech of a person, thereby identifying the start of cognitive damage or a psychotic episode.

For 2.5 years, an automatic learning algorithm assessed quarterly speech samples of 34 adolescents at high risk of psychosis, identifying with absolute precision 5 individuals who would have developed a psychosis; the algorithm proved to be much more accurate than clinical assessments[72].

[71] Bergenstal R.M., Klonoff D.C., Garg S.K., et al. "Threshold-based insulin-pump interruption for reduction of hypoglycemia", *N Engl J Med* 2013;369(3):224-232.

[72] Bedi G., Carrillo F., Cecchi G.A., et al. "Automated analysis of free speech predicts psychosis onset in high-risk youth", *NPJ Schizophr* 2015;1:15030.

A further example is linked to depression: a smartphone can identify negative thoughts underlying phrases, spoken or written in texts, such as: "it's all hopeless" and give forewarning of significant depressive episodes by identifying any increase in the frequency of such expressions and correlating them with a reduction in conversations with friends and increased time spent at home.

Automatic learning of natural language can provide benefits not only for the treatment of individuals but also for the entire population. For example, an algorithm that uses data extracted from more than 5 million Twitter messages[73] predicted the breakout of an influenza epidemic with extremely high precision, beating established methods such as analysis of searches made on the Web, in large part because it was able to correctly filter the messages sent by users who did not actually have influenza.

The availability of these algorithms and the ability to manage extensive groups of data that could not be analysed and interpreted in the past because of the inadequacy of existing processing tools represent significant new prospects for improving the treatment of the individual patient, by assuring them of the indisputable added value of artificial intelligence and the other technological developments that are now available. Levels of innovation to this extent are not without risks. The main risks are those connected with increasingly precise detection and registration of personal data collected in the sphere of daily life that can undermine the protection of privacy and create a potential opening for the exploitation of human vulnerability. Abuses of information about human health could be numerous.

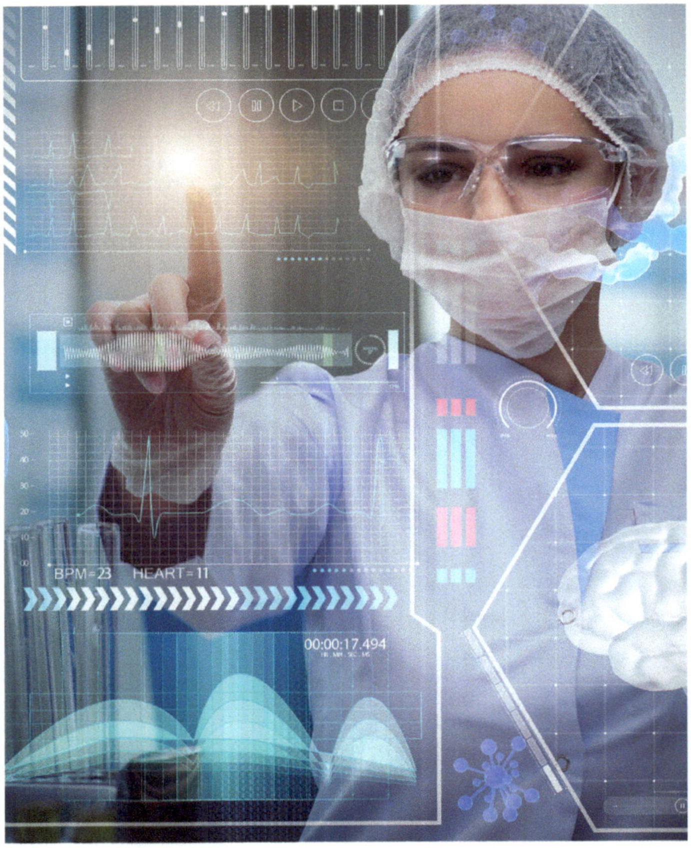

Precisely for this reason, a "balance" must be struck between the two intelligences: when automatic learning effectively becomes part of clinical practice, medicine is obliged to guarantee that this technology is exploited for social purposes in compliance with the ethical principles of the profession.

[73] Aramaki E., Maskawa S., Morita M. "Twitter Catches The Flu: Detecting Influenza Epidemics using Twitter", 2011.

Rigorous empirical validation of the new technologies compared with the clinical results is not exempt from the effort to create new ethical approaches to tackle the emerging dilemmas inherent in the use of automatic learning technologies in promoting health.

The Italian Medicines Agency is engaged in the issue. In a sector such as health, the challenge of minimising inappropriateness and ensuring sustainable reimbursement by the National Health Service is not merely important, it is vital for state budgets. Innovative information technology tools can enable patients to benefit from the most appropriate treatment available and to make the pathway that leads to the identification of the medicine to be used transparent, objective and traceable at any time.

The innovative schemes for access to medicines that the Italian Medicines Agency has proposed and the new detection methods using the monitoring registers are clearly good examples, acknowledged also at the European level[74] in the introductory speech of the Dutch Health Minister, Edith Schippers, as part of the event "Innovation for the benefit of the patients", organised during the Dutch Presidency of the Council of the European Union[75].

[74] AIFA. "AIFA come esempio in Europa per schemi innovativi di accesso ai farmaci" (*AIFA as an example in Europe for innovative schemes of access to medicines*). *AIFA* 2016.

[75] Darcy A.M., Louie A.L., Weiss Roberts L. "Machine Learning and the profession of medicine", *JAMA* 2016; 315(6):551-552; please see also notes 70, 71, 72 and 73.

4.2 Neuroscience and "systems biology": examples of modelling and advanced simulation in Alzheimer's disease

Two centuries ago, the cell was recognised as the structural and functional unit of organisms. Since then, knowledge about the smallest living structure has been enriched to an extraordinary degree, passing from the cellular description to the mapping of numerous genomes with the possibility of simulating certain complex biochemical reactions that are the result of activation of multiple and simultaneous molecular networks.

These are the results of so-called systems biology, an integrated approach that, for around 10 years, has been combining theoretical modelling with direct experimentation in a more systematic way. Theoretical or computational models provide knowledge on experimental observations; experiments can procure the data required for the creation of the models or confirm or deny their results. Many scientific discoveries and technological progress in other fields of engineering are based on models simulated on high-performance computers. This revolution is now beginning to touch the field of neurosciences and research on the brain, exciting the interest of researchers, companies, regulators, investors and payers. Recently, a number of concrete examples of the application of systems biology to the central nervous system were described[76]. It is clear that many neurological or psychiatric diseases such as schizophrenia or dementia, to mention but a few, are the result of interactions between multiple molecular networks and the surrounding environment. The models of many diseases of the human brain are so complex as to be impossible to reproduce with sufficient validity at the pre-clinical level in animals or in non-human primates. This limit has probably slowed down research and pharmacological development in the field of neurosciences so far, which has the highest rate of failure of new products.

Alzheimer-type dementia (AD) is perhaps the most striking example of the inadequacies of pre-clinical models; of around 300 products that have demonstrated activity in transgenic mice, not one new medicine has yet demonstrated significant efficacy in sick patients.

Modelling and simulation could constitute a valid alternative, especially when based on human clinical data and adequate sectorial expertise. The convergence of clinical and biological databases, however, requires complex calculation capacity ranging from bottom-up dynamic systems modelling to top-down probabilistic causal approaches. Various methodological frameworks developed for the modelling and analysis of complex multivariate data could be adapted to neurosciences in general and to AD in particular.

[76] Haas M., Stephenson D., Romero K. et al. "Big data to smart data in Alzheimer's disease: Real-world examples of advances modeling and simulation", *Alzheimer & Dementia* 2016;12(9):1022-1030.

Notwithstanding the enormous investments in identifying diagnostic or prognostic biomarkers, the gap between the exploratory research phase and their validation and integration in routine clinical practice remains wide. This is in part because conventional methods of analysis concentrate on the analysis of individual biomarkers, whereas most phenotypes of the disease do not arise from individual genes and proteins but from a complex network of molecular interactions.

An example of quantitative systems pharmacology (QSP) applied to Alzheimer's disease was recently qualified by the EMA[77] as an instrument with predictive value to be used in clinical trials.

In some cases, moreover, modelling and simulation have provided elements of support for the regulatory approval of a medicine under slightly different conditions, without the need for further clinical trials. In post-herpetic neuralgia, regulatory approval was granted for specific doses of gabapentin on the basis of sophisticated modelling of the response to exposure, using five clinical trials with different doses, without the need to conduct another clinical trial. The approved technical sheet explicitly states that "the pharmacokinetic/pharmacodynamics (PK/PD) modelling has provided evidence confirming efficacy at all doses". The antiepileptic oxcarbazepine was also approved as a monotherapy in children on the basis of advanced PK/PD modelling and subsequently confirmed in only one clinical trial. Recently, an advanced mechanism-based QSP was used to simulate the impact of recombinant human parathyroid hormone with reference to alternative dosage regimens. All this suggests that the regulatory agencies are increasingly interested in advanced multi-scale modelling and simulation over and above the more traditional PK/PD modelling.

There are clear and concrete fields of application of the knowledge acquired thanks to this integrated approach. One example is its use in support of programmes of discovery of new medicines (in terms of validation of the target and identification of the optimal modulation strategy for the selected target) in order to identify any population of responders for specific targets and to confirm clinical observations that can demonstrate relevant changes in the progression of the disease.

An essential prerequisite for the generation of usable knowledge is, however, the sharing of data in a standardised format. This is true for data from real-life situations and for data from clinical studies. Initiatives such as the Clinical Path Institute (C-Path) and the European Innovative Medicines Initiative are making progress in this area.

For certain qualitative relationships (for example, factors that determine clinical progression) deep analytical approaches based on advanced statistical methods are probably sufficient.

---

[77] http://www.ema.europa.eu/docs/en_GB/document_library/Regulatory_and_procedural_guideline/2013/10/WC500151309.pdf.

In this way, more complex quantitative questions can also be tackled with a better estimate of the progression of a placebo's trajectory. For more predictive and quantitative questions that are relevant for the actual discovery and development of medicines (that is, in which direction and how much must we therapeutically influence one or more biological processes in order to have a significant, measurable impact on the clinical phenotype in a specific patient population), the formalised integration of extensive expertise in the neurobiological domain seems to be a solution for better defining the causality between the various biological processes.

Moving from purely exploratory analyses to approaches that are, by their nature, more predictive is absolutely essential to support the development of new and improved therapeutic interventions. Combining data and advanced modelling algorithms with formalised expertise in the neurophysiological, clinical, imaging and neuropharmacological domains could be a breakthrough point in the research for new effective medicines for AD[76].

4.3 Quantity versus quality of the data and the "contamination" of technological innovation in the field of health

According to Wikipedia: "Big Data is the term used to describe a collection of data so extensive in terms of volume, velocity and variety as to require specific analytical methods and technologies for the extraction of value."

I have already had the opportunity to deal with the issue of Big Data in depth and their potential in the clinical and scientific field in the volume *Sustainable Innovation*. Around a year ago, I noted with interest the future scenarios prophesied by the former CEO of Google when he announced the progressive "disappearance of the Internet" in favour of its reincarnation in multiple devices and sensors that would populate the daily round of every one of us, collecting H24 data with the power of continuous interaction[78]. In effect, smartphones, iPads, wearable devices, sensors and now even "intelligent" tablets are already capable of recording hundreds of millions of bytes of information like streams of personal snapshots in time lapse. Some avant-garde analysts now argue that the "Internet of things" in the last 12 months (!) has been transformed into the "Internet of everything" and so into the "Internet of value". However, "the extraction of all this value" is not so clear cut. Nor is the storage, analysis, intersection and certification; in a nutshell, the restoration of sense to this boundless mass of data. All this has an aspect that is not trivial, and is influencing the strategic choices and marketing approaches of many companies, firstly, the pharmaceutical and IT companies that, not by chance, are setting up various partnerships for the management of Big Data in the field of the development of pro-health technologies and, in our field of interest, in the pharmaceutical sphere.

An example of this is the agreement signed in 2015[79] for clinical research on multiple sclerosis between Biogen and Google, or rather Verily, the subsidiary of the Mountain View group specialising in the medical and scientific field. The aim is to collect information on individuals with multiple sclerosis. From its analysis, it may be possible to identify the factors that contribute to manifestations of disease and, above all, the dynamics that regulate its progression in order to achieve the development of targeted medicines and treatments. Pharmaceutical companies do not have the calculation power necessary to process the data from such extensive analyses. But the major technological service companies do. Google, Apple, Microsoft and IBM, just to mention some significant examples of corporate dimensions, have been investing heavily in the health sector for some years.

[78] AIFA. "I Pazienti, la Salute Digitale e lo Io T" (*Patients, Digital Health and IoT*), *AIFA* 2015.

[79] Chen C. "Google, Biogen seek reasons for advance of multiple sclerosis". *Bloomberg* 2015.

Thanks also to the development of proprietary devices, they are in a position to "capture" the clinical data of patients. Google, for example, thanks to specific industrial agreements, is slowly acquiring expertise overseas in order to be able to take over the institutes responsible for the sustainability of federal welfare programmes. At least, this has been affirmed by the Vice President of Biogen's Strategic Development Division[80], after a year of collaboration with Google. "Payers," Adam Koppel recently stated during a Healthcare Conference at the Harvard Business School, "are becoming *de facto* information services companies." This statement is confirmed by the fact that, in the United States, health insurance companies are increasingly specialising in the collection and analysis of several different sets of real-life data on their patients in order to personalise welfare plans and possibly help patients to maintain in good health and thereby reduce the insurance risk.

Google does not even rule out the reverse process if, as Koppel remarks, it succeeds in reaching a position where it can replace the Centers for Medicare and Medicaid Services.

Beyond the interesting repercussions that this forecast could generate in the American health landscape, what gives us pause for thought as regulators is the profound interconnection of the technological world with that of health, which has emerged as one of the trends[81] in the medical science sector, at least for the period 2016–2018.

The need to "start from the patient", but from a different patient from the one understood up to now, from which to collect an enormous store of information in order to come up with solutions more targeted to their characteristics and personal needs, is at the basis of this shift of highly advanced information technology expertise in support of clinical research and policies of governance of healthcare expenditure. The data that measure the outcomes in patients in real time are of exceptional significance for the definition of personalised therapeutic plans and for the identification of truly effective reimbursement strategies.

For these reasons, we have invested in the monitoring registers. As a result, for example, it is possible to keep track in real time of various conditional reimbursement schemes for the same molecule with different therapeutic indications or the anti-HCV treatments launched in Italy, their number and therefore the opportunity to renegotiate new discounts with the manufacturing companies based on the results of the price-volume agreements. Or, with the capacity to optimise and recover economic resources from treatments that are not as effective as promised, by virtue of agreements to share the risk and conditional reimbursement mechanisms, savings of more than € 200 million were made in 2015 alone.

It is our duty to give notice of the policy changes that concern both research into new

[80] Keshavan M. "Biogen VP: Google wants to be a payer – and take over CMS", *MedCityNews* 2016.

[81] AIFA. "I trend del mondo della Medicina nel 2016" (*Trends in the world of Medicine 2016*), *AIFA* 2016.

medicines and the management of their economic sustainability because, in the institutional mandate of regulators/payers, these two purposes coexist, and this means that technological innovation must increasingly be used in the operational management of the Agency. This is the why, in recent years, the Italian Medicines Agency has supported a programme to boost its information technology systems that today, while still undergoing improvements, enable us to manage a continuous cycle of information concerning technical-scientific evaluations, those of a pharmaco-economic type and post-marketing analyses of actual clinical practice. We intend to use the data to feed a workflow that produces outcomes, to be reissued in their turn in the negotiating process, in order to generate meaning and steer the daily work towards increasingly better calibrated strategic choices.

In this unstoppable – and in parts revolutionary – progress in information technology, we hold a unique viewpoint that we do not regard as negotiable: that constituted by the privacy and individuality of the patient and the new responsibilities arising from taking charge of millions of "data generators", validating them and certifying their value.

4.4 The uncertain certainty of (im)precision medicine

We have already been able to explore the issue of precision medicine and to question the degree of accuracy that the new diagnostic pathways that arise from it manage to ensure, such as to provocatively describe it as potentially de-personalised[82]. The term that identifies a so-called "-omic" science seems solemnly charged with responsibility; but it risks attributing to it an almost absolute level of efficiency and certainty that we do not feel is shared by everyone. In reality, the exact opposite seems true, at a time when the precision of the genome actually unveils a plethora of so many variables that it is open to multiple interpretations, based on which the treatment pathway valid for each individual patient is "cut out". In this process, the key role belongs to the doctor and to those called upon to assess all the possible solutions with regard to the scientific rigour and the ability to replicate the results, and, not least, the wishes of the patient.
All the new diagnostic and information extraction techniques need to be profitably correlated with traditional clinical predictors. Oncology comes to mind, the branch in which precision medicine is mostly applied. The genomic tests on tumours must not replace traditional methods that identify their extent, degree and nodal status. For example, some studies on mutations in gene expression of breast cancer have certainly provided precious indications on the risk of relapse but no direct evidence on the efficacy or otherwise of specific treatments. They are studies of great scientific value because they assess the quality over time of the prognostic forecast derived from precision medicine techniques and concretely measure the certainty of the data, producing clinically valid results, but they are also fundamental studies; therapeutic choices cannot and must not be disregarded because it is not possible yet to be so certain of the molecular mechanism[83].
The greatest challenge is to succeed in personalising treatments based on the characteristics of each patient when the latter changes from one to many/everyone; in other words, framing these new diagnostic and prognostic tests in a statistically and clinically rational approach that produces reliable results.
This will be much more challenging in the near future when the range of variables to be considered reaches staggering proportions. The decisions on therapies are also influenced by the knowledge derived from the most advanced gene sequencing methods and, once a disease has been diagnosed, by all the possible prognostic analyses of the

[82] AIFA. "Terapie (s)personalizzate e il futuro della Medicina" [*(De)personalised therapies and the future of medicine*], AIFA 2015.
[83] Hunter D.J. "Uncertainty in the era of precision medicine", *N Engl J Med* 2016;375:711-713.

-omic disciplines. Knowing how to rationally and efficiently weigh up all these variables will also depend on how these data are presented, on categorisation of the risk and on the communication methods by which this information is then transferred directly to the patient, that is, the ultimate decision-maker.
It will be the patient who will be faced with numerous dilemmas with an insufficient degree of technical knowledge that clinicians and regulators must succeed in boosting by always responding responsibly and adequately to the classic age-old question: "What would you do in my place, doctor?".

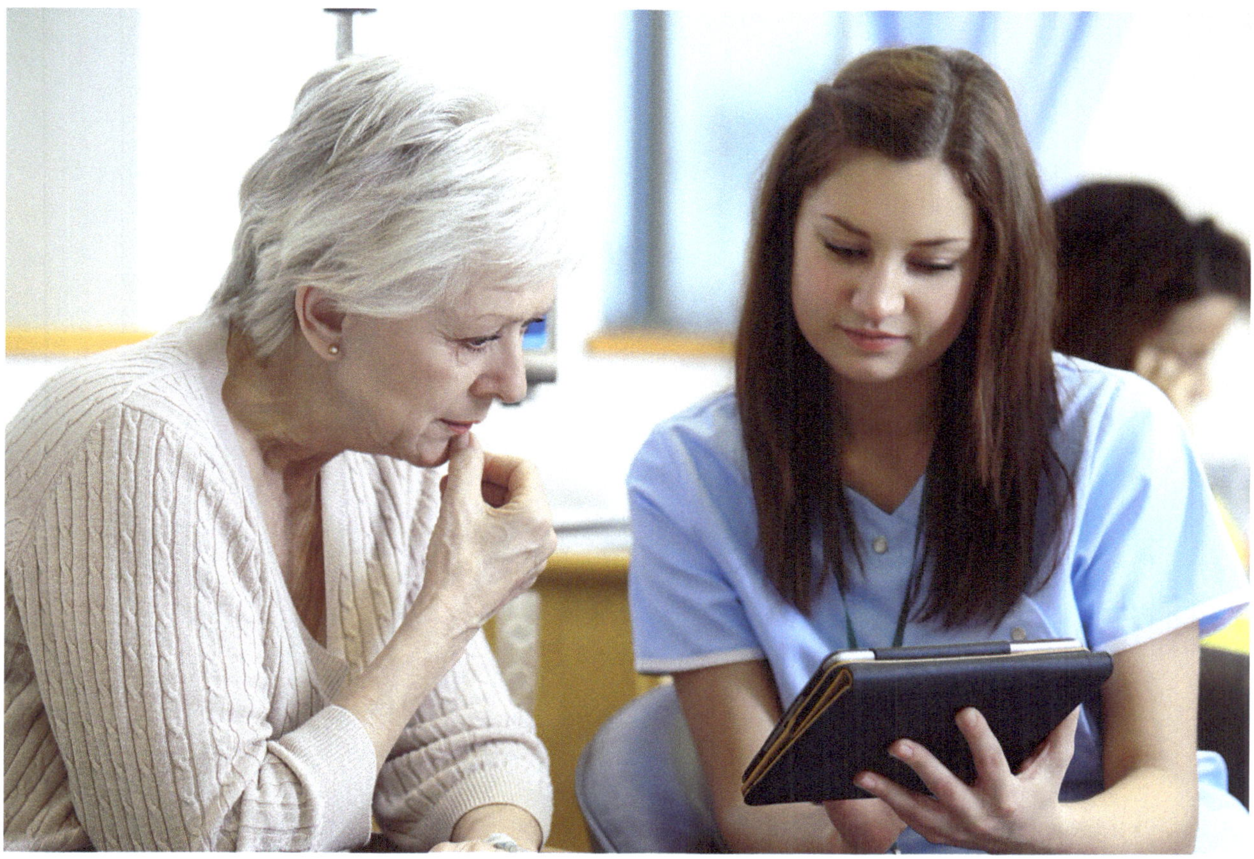

4.5 Digital technology at the service of health: a path to reduce costs and encourage the development of personalised medicine and "made-to-measure" medicines

Digital technology could provide effective solutions for many challenges that the health systems must tackle in the coming years, from the ageing of the population to the increase in costs of chronic diseases and the constant pressure on public health budgets.

The growing interest in the application of digital technologies in the health sphere is laying the foundations for a convergence of expertise and professionalism that, in respect of the dignity and rights of the person and with their willing and active involvement, has the potential to produce benefits for global health and health systems but also for the progress of knowledge and economic development.

We have already referred in previous pages to a sector undergoing strong expansion, for example, in the area of the so-called wearable devices, capable of detecting, storing and transmitting vital parameters (for example, heartbeat, oxygen saturation, breathing rate) measured in real time and, in certain cases, checking when determined thresholds are exceeded and generating alarm signals.

As in every segment of an emerging market, the prospects for wearable electronic devices currently present various factors of uncertainty. The market for products for the general public (general consumer wellness) is in rapid expansion, mobilising growing interest on the part of various public and private stakeholders, especially concerning the data generated by the latter. One very promising sector is that of wearable or perimeter devices and sensors for medical use (medical grade), which have the potential to deal with a number of serious problems for health systems worldwide but also favouring patient empowerment and the transition to personalised medicine.

In the United States, the FDA classifies wearables in the same way as medical devices, from class I (simple devices without potential risk) to class III (complex devices, with possible risk factors for patients). These new devices could have a significant impact on the health results and the costs of diseases such as diabetes, cardiovascular diseases, epilepsy, obesity, COPD, depression, dementia and Alzheimer's or Parkinson's disease.

These devices, together with mobile applications and other software, bring a predictive capacity that puts patients and healthcare operators in a position to identify early signals of disease or prevent flare-ups. Moreover, by generating a continuous flow of data in real life, they make speedy therapeutic adjustments possible, allowing monitoring of results in support of health policy or reimbursement decisions and incentivise changes in lifestyle to improve the overall effectiveness of interventions. They can also contribute to steering the processes of research and development and therapeutic interventions towards truly personalised medicine.

In order for these tools to become a pillar of health systems, providing all parties (payers, regulators, patients, companies, financial backers, researchers in the field of life sciences and new technologies) with a proposal of "real value" able to improve the health results, questions must be tackled such as the development costs, the usability, the security of the data, privacy, involvement of the patient, the role of the doctor and new methods of doctor-patient interaction.

In order to realise their remarkable potential, these devices must overcome a series of legal, regulatory, technical, practical and cultural barriers. A collaborative and widespread approach will therefore be necessary for the integration of wearables into the main flow of healthcare services but also among the instruments in support of the research and development of new molecules.

If these instruments, including the most advanced and futuristic ones, will soon be available and accessible on a large scale and if the data are shared and made available to the medical-scientific community in an open way and free of charge, it will be a significant step forward in diagnostics and the development of medicines. It will lay the foundation for improving the involvement of patients in the management of their diseases and the medicines with which they are treated.

Moreover, conditions will be created for an improved and more rational allocation of public resources to health, an indispensable prerequisite in order to guarantee to all citizens, under conditions of economic sustainability, the treatments they need, including innovative high-cost ones[84].

[84] "The hype and the hope: the journey from consumer to medical-grade wearables", *Pharmaphorum* 2016; Edney A., Chen C. "Big Pharma hands out fitbits to collect better personal data", *Bloomberg* 2015.

5. Change as a shared responsibility

5.1 Health research in Italy: opportunities for investment and relaunching the country's system

5.2 The value of "less is more" in the rationalisation of therapeutic treatments

5.3 "Miracle cures": the responsibility of information and the threat of "deregulation"

5.4 Rare diseases. The role of patients, the commitment of the regulator

5.1 Health research in Italy: opportunities for investment and relaunching the country's system

Quality health research, in addition to producing benefits for the health of citizens, is the engine of knowledge, innovation and development and contributes to the social, economic and cultural well-being of the country. Health costs are increasing rapidly everywhere in the world, but a large percentage of the expenditure sustained by governments is not productive (up to 30% in the United States, based on a report published a few years ago in the *New England Journal of Medicine* and in the *Journal of the American Medical Association*[85]). Quality research could generate new solutions to health needs, encouraging a more efficient allocation of health budgets.

It is for these reasons that making Italy one of the main players in health research in Europe would be an ambitious but very stimulating challenge and one within the reach of our country. Especially after Brexit, which is expected to be a hard Brexit, the roles freed up in the field of life sciences by the United Kingdom become a tempting opportunity for continental countries that want to snap them up.

Giving greater impetus to research by attracting investments from abroad and guaranteeing new resources for the National Health Service, however, means, above all, guaranteeing reliability and efficiency, anticipating the changes, relying on innovations, making full use and sharing the enormous mass of health data currently available thanks to the large digital databases; all things that Italy seems potentially to have but that it struggles to exploit due to the political and bureaucratic fetters that slow down – if not actually obstruct – the desirable critical independence and judgement of the technical and scientific institutions. Today, at the global level, most of the resources invested in research do not improve healthcare assistance or the health of the population because the current system generates enormous waste. Better management of the resources allocated to research is therefore a basic requirement. The ethical and economic financial profiles in this field are closely related.

The waste of resources, in addition to discouraging private investment and squandering public funds, is actually reflected in damage in terms of patient's health, generating widespread distrust in the capacity of the scientific community to systematically and efficiently use the results of the studies conducted[86]. All parties can contribute to improving these results but it is necessary to work in collaboration in order to define methods, times and strategies.

[85] Berwick D.M., Hackbarth A.D. "Eliminating waste in US healthcare", *JAMA* 2012;307(14): 1513-6.; Blumenthal D., Stremikis K., Cutler D. "Healthcare spending - a giant slain or sleeping?", *N Engl J Med* 2013;369:2551-2557; http://healthaffairs.org/healthpolicybriefs/brief_pdfs/healthpolicybrief_82.pdf.

[86] Moher D., Glasziou P., Chalmers I., et al. "Increasing value and reducing waste in biomedical research: Who's listening?", *Lancet* 2015;387:1573-1586.

In the specific field of pharmaceutical research, the Italian Medicines Agency has acted on various fronts in recent years, not just at the national level. Scientific and HTA consultancy to companies in the initial phases of the development of a medicine come to mind. Irrespective of what some Taliban think of the regulatory world, which is, however, provided on the individual level or through dilapidated foundations or private institutes, always ready to provide the same type of consultancy, early dialogue between the regulatory agencies and industry can reduce the margin of error in designing trials, encouraging a successful outcome of the registration process, and making medicines that prove to be truly innovative in less time and at lower cost.

In order to guarantee access to these medicines by assuring their economic sustainability, it is vital to identify and manage a national system to assess the efficacy, safety and the economic, ethical and social impact of technologies of health (HTA), with responsible participation of all the parties involved in various ways.

A priority objective is the relaunch of independent research, able to intercept health needs, steer health planning and contribute to the sustainability of the National Health Service. Thanks to independent research, it is indeed possible to study those populations neglected by the search for profit, resolve the uncertainties about medicines on the market, analyse the incidence of adverse events on large populations, and improve prescriptive appropriateness and adherence to treatments.

Great results, however, require synergy of intent and shared strategies: greater involvement of the patient, laid down, among other things, by the new European Regulation on clinical trials to be adopted from 2018, a growing and increasingly profitable PPP, and integration of private research with that funded by the state, which does not replace but integrates and completes industrial research.

5.2 The value of "less is more" in the rationalisation of therapeutic treatments

The responsibility to succeed and ensure the right to treatment and, at the same time, the sustainability of the system is also derived from rational choices that accompany prescriptive appropriateness in a relationship of shared knowledge between the doctor and the patient on the most suitable therapeutic pathways.

"The most effective treatment can sometimes be ' non-treatment'", K.B. Thomas wrote in the *British Medical Journal* as far back as 1978. The Portsmouth GP introduced the concept of "therapeutic illusion" for the first time, the overestimated capacity perceived by clinicians of succeeding in identifying the most effective therapeutic treatments and in feeling enthusiastic and immediately conclusive in the approach to their patients' disorders even in cases of uncertain diagnosis[87]. The tendency to discern causality between events, although not objectively possible, is, actually, an innate characteristic shared by all of us. Psychologists define it as the "illusion of control", as reported by David Casarett, a doctor at the University of Pennsylvania and author of an in-depth article on this issue published in the *New England Journal of Medicine*[88]. This is a phenomenon with various shades and contexts: for example, it is the gambler's sense of invincibility when performing propitiatory rites before rolling the dice that influences his everyday life. Or, the thrilling attitude of volunteers in an experiment to solve a simple problem like turning on a light on a panel, unaware that the light turns on and off purely by chance.

The consequences of such an inclination in clinical practice are not trivial and very often combine in a proliferation of futile examinations and prescriptions, the so-called "over-treatment" that, for some years, we have tried to rationalise with targeted awareness campaigns. "Too much medicine"[89] from the *BMJ* and "Choosing Wisely"[90] launched by the foundation of the American Board of Internal Medicine (ABIM Foundation) are two examples of initiatives that promote a reduction in redundant interventions in medicine through the dissemination of recommendations, updates of the literature, the involvement of scientific societies and, above all, the patients themselves. Often it is not only the therapeutic illusion that influences the choices of healthcare operators; other external pressures, such as those from the sick or their families, contribute to overestimated prescriptions and excessive examinations.

---

[87] Thomas K.B. "The consultation and the therapeutic illusion", *Br Med J* 1978;1(6123):1327-1328.

[88] Casarett D. "The science of choosing wisely - overcoming the therapeutic illusion", *N Engl J Med* 2016;374:1203-1205.

[89] http://www.bmj.com/too-much-medicine.

[90] http://www.choosingwisely.org/.

This close relationship between doctor and patient was well illustrated by Thomas almost 40 years ago, when he defined the doctor as a "powerful therapeutic agent *per se*" or "the most used drug in general medicine" and we have written recently on this[91]. The expectation generated in the surgery before a visit is ambivalent; there is the expectation of a diagnosis and a treatment on the part of the patient and the unconscious awareness of having to dispense a prescription on the part of the doctor, dictated by a natural wish to be able to treat the patient. An unjustified enthusiasm for pharmacological treatment on the part of both, as Thomas defines it, is often not followed by an equal concern over its results.

Therapeutic illusion can, in fact, also be complicit in an overestimate of the benefits associated with a particular treatment, which is often reinforced in the case of positive outcomes that are actually entirely random. Sometimes there is a tendency on the part of doctors to take into consideration only those results that confirm the wisdom of their therapeutic choice, ignoring those suggesting the contrary. A proper corrective in these cases could lie in critically seeking other reasons for a clinical improvement and not being limited to deeming it a direct consequence of prescription of an effective treatment[88]. Taking account of this human attitude and learning to recognise and manage it is a good approach for the application of evidence-based medicine. However, to think of reducing ineffective over-treatment by simply countering the effects of the therapeutic illusion would be to fall victim of a vicious circle.

There is the need for a strategy, subject to appropriate future research, that objectively and with new instruments rationalises the excessive treatment of patients. Training is required in the schools of specialisation on the issue of the therapeutic illusion and the dissemination of a medical "culture" that involves not only clinicians but also the rest of the actors included in the treatment process[88]. A patient-centred and, at the same time, evidence-informed approach balances special attention on the individual patient and their needs with constant comparison of the therapeutic choices and with the broadest and most up-to-date scientific evidence. A personalised method is also required on the part the healthcare operator who, thanks to the recommendations and guidelines and awareness campaigns promoting the responsible recourse to health treatments, manages to choose wisely by reviewing their convictions, assessing the evidence and applying heuristic criteria objectively and rigorously.

[91] Corbellini G., Pani L. *Prescrivere Valore. Storia e Scienza dei farmaci che ci fanno vivere più a lungo e meglio* [*Prescribing value. History and science of medicine that help us live longer and better].* EDRA-LSWR, 2017, Milan.

5.3 "Miracle cures": the responsibility of information and the threat of "deregulation"

The so-called "medical tourism" has existed for many years but, in recent years, has seen an extraordinary evolution thanks to globalisation, the spread of the Internet and the ease of low-cost travel. But not just that. The phenomenon is not necessarily negative. It may simply be the result of a search for a standard treatment at lower cost or with shorter waiting times, or a treatment that is already well-regulated but perhaps less accessible elsewhere. It is not rare, however, to encounter stories of patients who undertake long and difficult journeys to reach countries with weak or non-existent regulatory systems in the search for "miracle treatments". Stories that hit the headlines.

In recent years, for example, "stem cell tourism" has taken flight by people driven by the mirage of stem cell-based treatments, often untested treatments that promise a cure-all for everything from neurodegenerative diseases to diabetes, from paralysis to autism, with almost zero regulatory control; patients with fatal diseases but also people who are readily disposed to spend considerable sums to cure disorders. Often, patients seeking new "cures" do not even want to know which substances will be administered, whether or not evidence exists of their efficacy or whether the risks of a treatment are monitored, deciding to undergo ineffective treatments, sometime dangerously and, in the final analysis, also costly, driven by astonishing promises found on the Web.

Part of the blame for this superficiality often lies in the excessive simplification of the "discoveries" in the biomedical field and, above all, their exaggeration by the newspapers, radio and TV, that often end up creating false hopes and bitter disappointment for patients and their families.

The key to the phenomenon could lie in the Latin phrase *argumentum ad novitatem*: the attraction of the new. It is the "new", the novelty, which is, of itself, an extremely alluring term, amplified by the means of information, especially in the field of medicine and therapeutic innovations with an aspect of potential commercial development.

In the case of stem cell-based therapies, the demand has been steered by the enormous media coverage of the issue, with articles that often do not even distinguish between the various types of stem cells, and that communicate excessive optimism over the prospects for the short-term success of these therapies. Enthusiasm that seems undiminished even when setbacks occur, such as, for example, the interruption of the pioneering experiments of the Geron Corporation regarding a therapy with embryonic stem cells for the treatment of spinal cord injuries.

An analysis[92] published by two Canadian researchers in *Science Translation Medicine* under the title "The media hullabaloo on stem cells", studied the image of translational research provided by the main newspapers in Canada, the United States and the United Kingdom. The results demonstrate that, in most of the articles, the issue was treated with excessive optimism, contributing to the generation of unfounded hopes both on the times and the real availability of certain therapies. The two authors of the article, Kaline Kamenova and Timothy Caulfield, concluded that the great optimism of the media can effectively contribute to feeding unrealistic expectations among patients for dubious treatments still a long way from clinical application; scientists also play their part, used by the media to obtain authoritative statements that, in many cases, provide unreliable time indications regarding the availability of the treatments.

According to R. Alta Charo, lecturer in law and bioethics at the University of Wisconsin, who recently published an article on the issue in the *New England Journal of Medicine*, genetic editing, which has given encouraging results in trials recently, is also at risk of media sensationalism and could trigger a new wave of medical tourism. Genetic editing has also been well-known since the 1990s with ZFNs (zinc finger nucleases) and TALENs (transcription activator-like effector nucleases); the new CRISPR technique (clustered regularly interspaced short palindromic repeats)-Cas, introduced in 2012, has led to increased attention from the press and TV, fed by the controversy over the potential manipulation of human embryos and enthusiasm for the range of possible uses of somatic cells.

The CRISPR-Cas9 technique was described by *Science* as the most important discovery of 2015. After the news of the interruption of the progression of Duchenne dystrophy in an animal model, headlines appeared in the main daily newspapers and scientific disclosure websites such as "Genetic editing offers hope for the treatment of Duchenne muscular dystrophy". So it was in the case of the promising results obtained from the ZFN technique in the attempt to cure leukaemia in a young girl when headlines appeared such as "Genetic editing technique treats leukaemia in a young girl". Headlines like these inevitably convey messages of hope that reinforce the impression that treatments are available and lead patients to believe that the new therapies are at a really advanced level. It should not then be surprising if patients, reading often misleading headlines, think that the treatments are already available. Not everyone reads beyond the headline.

Moreover, this leads to a growing misperception of the slowness of the regulatory procedures, even though the regulatory authorities are introducing more and more ways of rapidly approving and providing access to experimental therapies.

[92] Kamenova K., Caulfield T. "Stem cell hype: Media portrayal of therapy translation", *Science Translational Medicine* 2015;7(278):278 ps4.

It would be wise to adopt measures now to guard against this possible phenomenon. A concerted information effort by researchers, companies and operators is required to find the thin line between the right to hope on the part of patients and media sensationalism, and to succeed in explaining that the best way to find safe and effective treatments is only through careful clinical experimentation and the evaluation of those treatments. Journalists and scientific editors should ensure that the articles and the associated headlines are written appropriately; scientists should be careful about the messages that are disseminated, and the regulatory authorities should collaborate among themselves and with patient associations in order to develop credible and accurate sources of information and work to draw up responsible research protocols and patient monitoring measures.

5.4 Rare diseases. The role of patients, the commitment of the regulator

For public decision makers, and so also for the regulatory agencies, the patient's perspective has a precious value, even more so when the pathological condition is not common and concerns people of geographical areas, genetic profiles, economic, cultural and social conditions that are often profoundly different. Networking, furnishing representation, contributing to the advancement of research and treatments is the best way to construct adequate pathways of healthcare continuity, indispensable in the overall management of a disease, and to accelerate access to new therapies.

For a long time, this centrality of the sick person was not acknowledged; they were considered the final recipients and not the leading figures in the process of research and treatment. In recent years, that trend has changed and the regulatory agencies have displayed growing interest in involving the patient, especially those with rare diseases.

Living with a rare disease is not[93], in fact, a rare condition. It seems a paradox, but it is not, when it is realised that the number of currently known and diagnosed rare diseases oscillates between 7000 and 8000 and tends to increase with scientific advances and especially with progress in genetic research. This does not concern just a few sick people but millions in Italy and tens of millions throughout Europe (in our country, the estimate is 1–2 million and 70% are children of paediatric age)[94].

Suffering from a rare disease must not be synonymous with isolation, dejection and mistrust. To avoid the knife-edge of desperation, it is therefore necessary to come together, to build bridges, to make voices heard, and be ready for discussion, committed to sharing common pathways.

The main expectation of the sick person lies in the discovery of new and effective treatments. However, research takes time, marked by a series of stages that ensure its transparency and scientific value, averting, in most cases, those false hopes that harm the sick person more than the lack of a treatment. For this reason, the Italian Medicines Agency has always argued that research must follow its course and not undergo the emotional influences of the day, and that, in this journey, early collaboration with those who develop a medicine enables the times and costs to be optimised and access to effective treatment to be accelerated.

Rare diseases are often not among the priority objectives of industrial research. Recruiting a sufficiently representative patient population to produce evidence of value is, in fact, more difficult and costly than for diseases with high prevalence; and when the process is

[93] In the European Union, the threshold established to define a rare disease is 5 cases in 10,000 people.

[94] Rete Orphanet Italia, http://www.orpha.net/consor4.01/www/cgi-bin/?lng=IT.

concluded successfully, the revenues are not always sufficient to repay the capital invested. An appeal can be made to the social responsibility of the pharmaceutical companies but it is also necessary to create conditions that make this line of research more attractive and provide instruments capable of placing value on real innovation.

A very important front, especially in the field of rare diseases, is independent research, which, in recent years, has produced significant results in the treatment of rare diseases in various therapeutic areas. Between 2012 and 2015, the EMA approved 57 new orphan medicines, of which 15 were in 2015: 6 anti-cancer medicines, 5 for the alimentary tract and the metabolism, 2 for the nervous system, 1 for ophthalmology and 1 antifungal medicine. Italy has developed consolidated institutional sensibility to the treatment of patients with rare diseases. From 2010 to the present day, the expenditure on orphan medicines has more than doubled, exceeding €1.2 billion (equal to around 6.8% of the total pharmaceutical expenditure). Under the profile of access to pharmacological treatments, in our country, people with rare pathologies, under certain conditions, can obtain access to medicines not yet authorised at the central level, making use of appropriate legislative instruments[95].

In recent years, in order to accelerate the availability of orphan medicines, those of exceptional therapeutic relevance or important to hospitals, the period for notification by the Italian Medicines Agency for classification and reimbursement by the National Health Service has been reduced from 180 to 100 days. Furthermore, specific economic protection is provided for the owners of orphan medicines that, in the event that hospital expenditure overshoots the ceiling, are exempt from compensation. In application of the new discipline, the Italian Medicines Agency has defined the criteria for drawing up a list of orphan medicines, on the basis of which the medicines for which the legal benefits apply can be identified.

In the near future, other targeted and personalised medicines, the outcome of progress in genomics, biotechnologies and nanotechnologies, will also impinge on the vast area of rare diseases. The road towards these therapies for the sick will be complex, however, in the light of the high costs that impact on health budgets. In pursuing this direction, the contribution of patients will be increasingly decisive.

An informed and participating patient is also a person who believes that quality of life is not a concept that is incompatible with their disease and who is committed to making their existence of benefit to themselves and others.

[95] The Law 648 of 1996, which allows the use of a medicine on a national basis; the Law 326 of 2003, article 48 (AIFA fund); the Ministerial Decree 8 May 2003 (compassionate use); the Law 94 of 1988 (formerly Di Bella Law).

6. Innovations in healthcare: the role of the pharmacist

6.1 Changes underway: the scenario of reference

Before we can speak of innovation and change, we must make a distinction, and not just a semantic one, between certain terms that are often confusing or overlapping, such as invention, innovation and dissemination. Invention can be defined as the genesis, often unexpected or casual, of a new idea, a new device or product, a scientific development or a technological novelty. The inventor, in spite of what may be believed, is rarely driven by economic or competitive reasons but rather by the intellectual "challenge" represented by the specific problem to be solved.

Innovation is the actual realisation of the invention by means of a new product or production process as well its commercial exploitation. Not all inventions are translated into innovations and many innovations are not derived directly from inventions. Indeed, the term has a plurality of meanings; innovation is synonymous with the adoption of a new organisational model, the creative combination of existing knowledge, the opening up to new markets, adaptation of the offer taking account of changes in demand, the introduction of a new production method. It was the famous Austrian economist Joseph Schumpeter, speaking about innovation, who coined the expression "creative destruction" – almost 80 years ago – underling how the innovative process can have such an intense impact on certain sectors that the companies that belong to it are obliged to evolve, on pain of extinction[96]. We use the term "dissemination" to describe the adoption of an innovation by businesses and consumers.

The world, at least in certain technological spheres, is now evolving in an exponential way and, as always when this happens, technology contributes to the transformation of habits, from the fire to the wheel, from the engine to electricity, from the telephone to the Internet. Nevertheless, the speed with which technological changes are disseminated among users has increased in recent decades. These changes will be particularly evident in the health world and in the future of healthcare assistance, and although, to many, it may seem like something distant and remote, this revolution will involve everyone first hand.

Transformations will inevitably be promoted by technological progress in the field of information technology, the development of machine learning, nanotechnologies and electronics, mostly but not exclusively, in the sphere of sensors.

The future of healthcare assistance will proceed in parallel with our own future. Its success will depend on our capacity to coherently work towards the creation of systems

[96] Schumpeter J.A. *Business cycles: a theoretical, historical, and statistical analysis of the capitalist process,* Northwestern University, 1939.

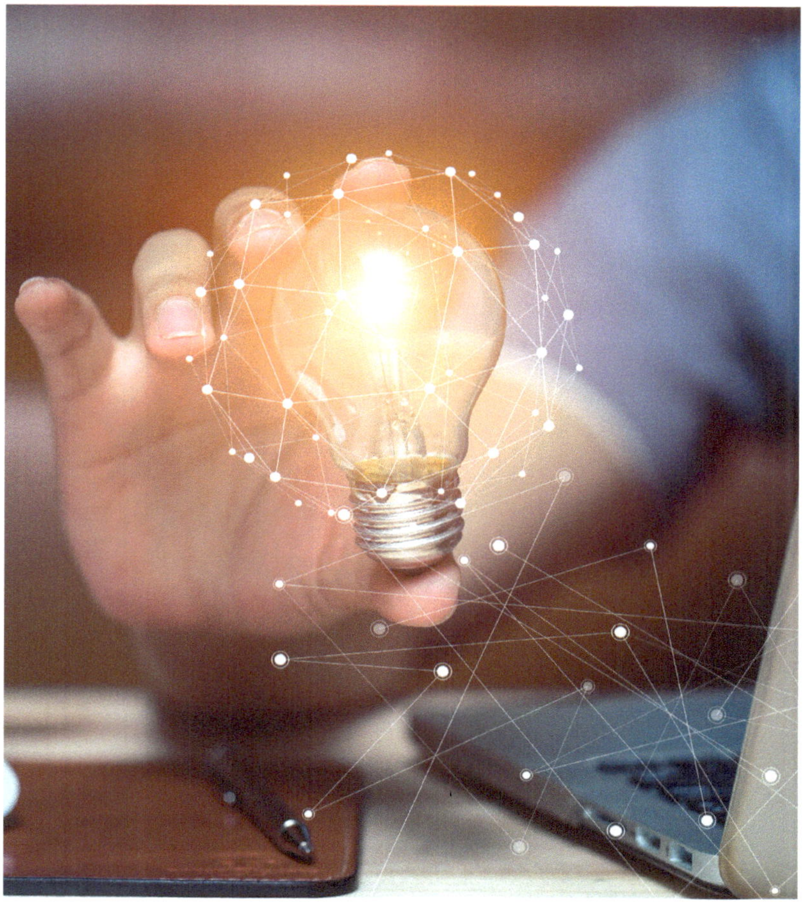

of individual and social organisation that are focused on the patient.
It will be a future where it will be possible to prevent illnesses before they have to be treated, where the key word will be simplification, where information will follow the patients wherever they go in order to ensure more convenient treatments that meet individual needs, where waste is reduced in tandem with an increase in productivity.
The health system of the future will not base its success on the volume of transactions (volume-based) but rather on the quality of the service offered (value-based); informed and constantly updated patients will play an active part in the treatment process, weighing up choices and decisions on the basis of their needs, and the so-called payers of health services will act as "coaches", promoting healthier lifestyles. Many of the barriers that still divide medicine into silos that do not communicate with each other will be knocked down, and this will enable all the stakeholders to develop new forms of organisation, sharing risks and results. Providers, payers, governments and suppliers will, in this way, be able to coordinate the resources available in a more efficient way in order to offer better services.
In the following paragraphs, some of the main developments and innovations that will accompany us in the coming years are presented.

6.2 Treatment after 2030: the advent of the home-spital

It could just be a provocation, or the vision of the near future. Melanie Walker, neurologist, lecturer at Washington University, Vice President of the World Economic Forum's Future Council and consultant to the World Bank, argues that, starting from 2030, most treatments that were previously administered in hospitals will be carried out directly at home. According to her, in 2030 prevention will be the basis of the world of medicine; the increase in safety at every level will enable reduction in the percentage of traumas, factories will be populated by robots and the number of road accidents will fall dramatically thanks to cars that drive themselves, with the consequence of fewer broken arms and legs.

The treatment of pathologies of cardiological origin will be more problematic; due to the epidemic of the metabolic syndrome in recent decades, heart attacks and strokes will remain the leading cause of death in advanced societies and, in these cases, prevention will also play a major role. To highlight the importance of preventive action, consider the data from the Eurostat surveys, which report that 1 death in 5 in the European Union is due to a heart attack or a stroke, specifically around 644,000 deaths were caused by heart attacks and around 433,000 by strokes[97].

Wearable monitoring devices, which are already a reality, will communicate data on our heart rate and blood pressure in real time to doctors, and implanted neural sensors in the brain will be able to rapidly and safely diagnose imminent potential disorders.

For pathologies of lesser importance and with less impact on the organism, it will be possible to have remote dialogue with the doctor; for more serious disorders, it will be possible to visit small, highly specialised facilities that will gradually replace larger and more costly hospitals.

Scanning the patient with technologies that will enable the combination of radiology, magnetic resonance and spectroscopy (without having to resort to biopsies), will provide doctors with all the details on the metabolic functions of the patients. There will no longer be any wait for organ donations because these will be produced by the latest-generation 3D biological printers, on demand, obviously personalised to order for the individual patient. It seems like a delirious vision of the medicine of the future but, in reality, many of these things are already with us.

[97] Eurostat: *Causes of death in 2013*, 4 May 2016.

6.3 Humans and Big Data

Today Big Data is all we talk about. Less clear is what they are, how they are generated and managed and, above all, in what way they can be important for our healthcare.
To give an example of their definition, Big Data are data whose size and complexity requires the development of new technological solutions and new methodologies for their analysis. The mass of data is currently in the order of zettabytes[98], rapidly heading towards yottabytes, and this requires equivalent and adequate calculation powers. Big Data also represent the interrelation of data from potentially diverse sources, mostly unstructured, such as images, emails, GPS data, information taken from the social networks and so on. The creation of very fast systems is therefore necessary that are capable of interrelating these data in order to transform them into information that can be processed further.
It is forecast that, in the coming 5 years, and thereafter increasingly so, the healthcare world will be producing an enormous mass of data, from population registers, diseases and real-life use of medicines, laboratories, pharmacies, insurance companies, electronic medical records, instruments monitoring vital parameters and also from blogs and social media. This data melting pot is potentially a source of unique knowledge for scientists. However, the main problem is the difficulty in interpreting all this information using traditional analysis. The creation of an integrated database has become necessary, oriented to the collection of Big Data and their rapid interrogation in order to carry out fast statistical analyses that enable instruments to be developed in support of decisions and a system that enables analysis of the individual's clinical data in order to identify the best treatment from an economic and clinical point of view or to identify the people who require changes in lifestyle. Passing from individuals to society, the progress and spread of an epidemic can be monitored, allowing decision makers to take preventive and/or containment actions.
This is an approach that surpasses the traditional clinical method based on adopting treatment protocols depending on the diseases. The aim is to identify specific medicines and ad hoc treatment methods to be used by virtue of a specific method of manifesting the illness in a certain individual.

[98] 1 zettabyte = 1000^7 = 10^{21} byte = 1 sextillion bytes.

6.4 The new technologies: drones for delivering medicines

A drone is nothing other than an aircraft piloted remotely, characterised by the absence of a human pilot on board. Its flight is controlled by a computer on the aircraft under the remote control of a navigator or pilot.
In the collective imagination, when drones are discussed, panoramic filming and the possibility of taking photos from on high come to mind. In addition to the fun aspect, in most cases drones can be used for other purposes. They can be used in agriculture, for deliveries or surveillance. They are also extremely useful in cases of emergency, especially earthquakes and floods, because they are able to provide assistance to people in difficult conditions and allow rescues to be coordinated at best.
An innovative use of these aircraft could be delivering objects of all types, including medicines, directly to the home, in order to help the elderly and disabled or whoever requests them. The objective of this ambitious project is to rapidly deliver to anyone the treatment that they need at lower prices. Too often, it can happen that, in difficult situations or places, critical health products risk deteriorating or not reaching the people who urgently need them. Thanks to drones, it will be possible to make deliveries to remote and often inaccessible locations.
The delivery of a medicine would be broken down into various, correlated phases. On the day set for the delivery, the user receives a series of notifications that remind them to pick up the package. When the drone is near the location agreed for the delivery, a message is forwarded to the recipient so that they can best organise the pickup. By means of a GPS localizer, the aircraft positions itself with the utmost precision in the established location, at the same time telephoning the recipient and thereafter leaving the package on the ground. The recipient, after picking up the package, can send confirmation of the delivery through a smartphone or computer.
It can therefore be appreciated how the drone could be an extremely versatile means of transport, as well as being environmentally friendly, and could easily be used by those who provide e-commerce services. However, in addition to the numerous advantages, account must be taken of certain risks in delivering the service; in particular, operating solutions must be studied in the case of deliveries to the wrong person or when the recipient is absent, as well as protecting against thefts or acts of vandalism.
A critical aspect, which could be solved, for example, with the aid of telemedicine, as we will see later, is the lack of a professional of reference for the disclosure of the information required to take the medicines delivered correctly and to ensure the therapy is duly followed.

6.5 The new services in the pharmacy

In Italy, Legislative Decree 153/2009 and subsequent implementation decrees have changed the face of the pharmacy, introducing the "pharmacy of services", providing distribution of services and professional assistance to citizens, including through local pharmacies. The aim is always to ensure the best local assistance within the containment of the total health expenditure.
As stated in article 11 of the Law of 18 June 2009, no. 69: "The Government is delegated to adopt, [...] one or more legislative decrees aimed at identifying new services with strong socio-healthcare value delivered by public and private pharmacies as part of the National Health Service." These are the main new measures:

- Integrated home assistance: the community pharmacist will be called upon to collaborate with GPs to ensure and monitor the correct use of prescribed medicines for the purpose of encouraging adherence of the sick to the medical therapies.
- Preliminary analyses: diagnostic instruments that the citizen will use to keep the key values of their state of health under constant control will be available for preliminary analyses.
- Bookings of visits and specialist examinations: it will be possible to book visits and specialist examinations at public and affiliated private facilities. The citizen will also be able to pick up the findings and arrange payment of their share of the cost.
- Health education programmes and prevention campaigns to combat the main diseases.

In future, it will be appropriate to go beyond these new services, in particular exploiting the full potential offered by the new information technologies. Consider, for example, the fact that computers, with the aid of increasingly precise algorithms, have begun to recognise patterns rapidly and effectively, producing more accurate diagnostic hypotheses. Widely used instruments such as automated meters can rapidly analyse different types of blood cells, diagnosing malaria and leukaemia. By investing the equivalent of only US$1000, hospitals will soon be able to improve their computer systems with graphic processors that could increase the analysis capacity to as many as 260 million images a day.
Given the derisory costs and the simplicity of use of these instruments and considering the tendency towards delocalization and disintermediation, including in the health field, the question arises of why not carry out certain types of these analyses in pharmacies. In the case of moles, for example, artificial intelligence can distinguish the difference between

innocuous and potentially fatal blemishes to a sufficient degree of accuracy. Images collected in the databases can boost the machine learning process. The scanning of moles, as well as other types of cells, could be carried out in pharmacies and come to be considered a routine activity, leaving dermatologists much more time to specialise in other aspects of the discipline.

In the next sections, we discuss the preliminary analytical services that can be conducted in the pharmacy involving screening; activities delivered at the pharmacies and in the homes of patients by professionals such as nurses and physiotherapists; telemedicine and the use of social media and Whatsapp-type text messaging by pharmacies.

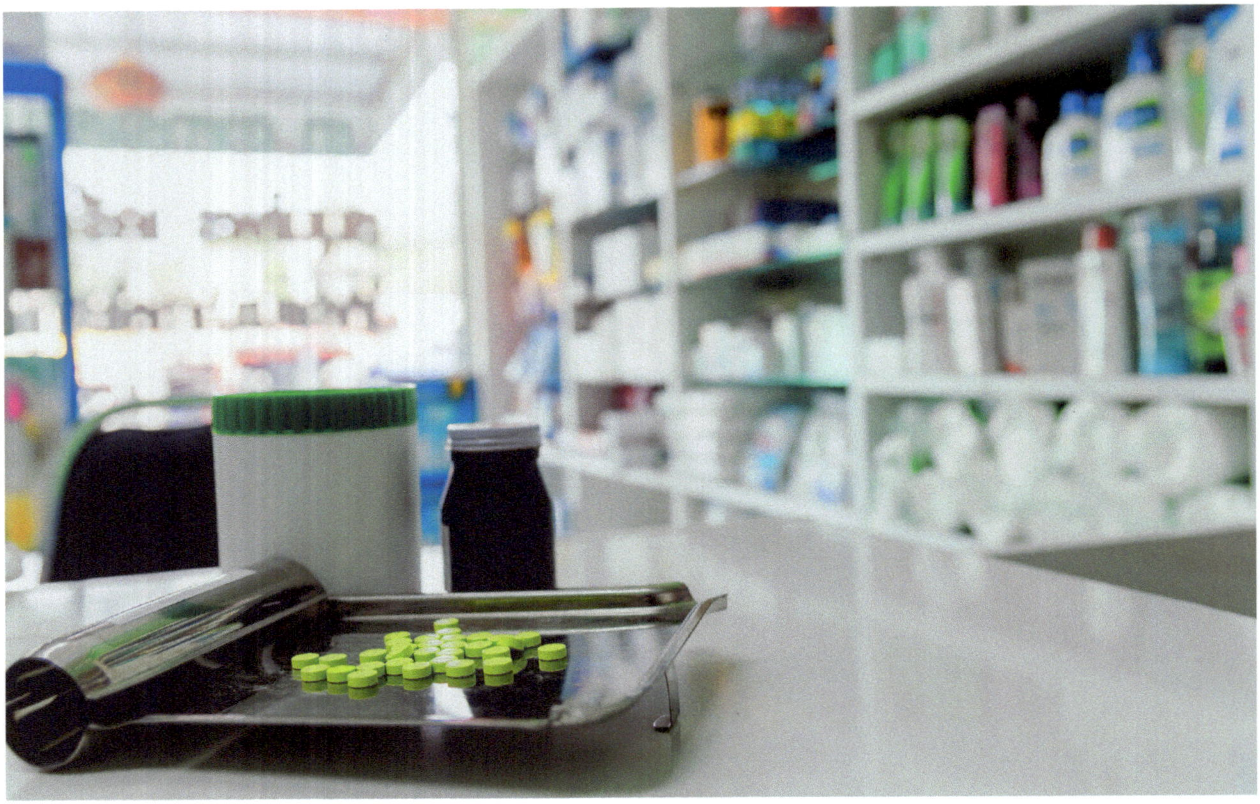

6.6 Screening in the pharmacy

We define screening as a strategy of generalised diagnostic investigations, used to identify an illness in a population at medium risk of an illness. Screening provides blanket medical examinations of the entire population in question that, by definition, does not yet display any symptoms or clinical signs of disease. This type of diagnostic procedure is a concrete opportunity for personal prevention.

As reported by the data from the National Screening Monitoring Centre, 13 million invitations were sent out in Italy in 2015 and slightly less than 6 million tests were carried out. Taking account of the increase in the number of tests compared with 2014 (+300,000), these numbers are certainly positive but there are huge margins for improvement. The gap between the Centre-North and South Italy is particularly significant.

The primary role of the pharmacy is confirmed in this context as the place where healthcare is delivered in the most immediate and accessible way for citizens. As recently underlined by the European Pharmacists Forum (EPF), "pharmacies can identify early the people most at risk, thereby enabling prompt action". It was also shown how it is possible "to use pharmacies to carry out the screening of diseases for which early intervention could lead to a containment of the costs"[99].

There are numerous tests that can be carried out directly in the pharmacy, including screening for atrial fibrillation, osteoporosis, venous insufficiency, as well as spirometry, oncological biomarkers in the DNA, for colorectal diseases and the prevention of strokes.

Automated screening for diabetic retinopathy has been receiving particular attention lately[100]. This disease, if detected in the initial phases, can be slowed significantly, limiting the damage to sight. With the increase in the diabetic population, there is an urgent need for automated screening of the disease and continuous monitoring. The instrument automatically analyses the images of the retinal fundus and collects the information from all the images, automatically generating a summary report. After a certain number of examinations, the instrument, by aligning the retinal images, is able to localize the presence of microaneurysms by analysing the dynamics over time, in order to evaluate the risk of rupture.

[99] *The role of the pharmacy in support of the health of citizens. White Book of the EPF and request for interventions.* European Pharmacists Forum (EPF), 2015.

[100] Common complication of diabetes is the main cause of sight loss in the working age population.

6.7 Professional services in the pharmacy

The Decree of 16 February 2010, published in the Official Gazette no. 90 of 19 April 2011, regulates the activities of healthcare operators in Italian pharmacies. The activities delivered at pharmacies and at the homes of patients must be carried out exclusively by nurses and physiotherapists in possession of the prerequisites.

A nurse in the pharmacy can: arrange the correct application of diagnostic-therapeutic prescriptions; offer support in the preliminary analytic determinations within the sphere of self-control (for example, glycaemia); perform intramuscular injection of medications; conduct activities concerning health education and participation in consulting programmes, including personalised programmes; take part in initiatives aimed at encouraging the adherence of the sick to the therapies.

On the prescription of GPs and primary care paediatricians, the physiotherapist can deliver the following professional services inside the pharmacy and at the patient's home: definition of a service programme for the aspects under their responsibility aimed at prevention, identification and meeting the needs for rehabilitation; therapeutic activities for functional re-education of motor, psychomotor, cognitive and visceral disabilities using manual, masso-therapeutical and occupational therapies; verification that the rehabilitation methodology implemented corresponds with the objectives of functional recovery.

6.8 Telemedicine

The "commissioning" of the immense functionality of information technology is indubitably one of the major opportunities and, at the same time, one of the major challenges facing all health systems, public or private, in the world. This type of technological innovation can contribute to a reorganisation of assistance, encouraging a shift of the main hub from the hospital to the locality through innovative assistance models that place the citizen at the centre and that facilitate access to the services within the country. A practical example of this evolution is telemedicine.

Telemedicine refers to a method of healthcare assistance service delivery through recourse to innovative technologies, especially those that concern information and communication technologies (ICT), in situations where the health professional and the patient (or two professionals) are not in the same place. Telemedicine transmits, in a secure way, medical information and data in the form of texts, sounds, images or other forms required for the prevention, diagnosis, treatment and subsequent control of patients[101].

In industrialised countries, telemedicine enables patients to receive treatment directly at home; in developing countries, it is used to overcome the barriers that reduce access to health services, including the lack of resources and the great geographical distances.

The benefits of telemedicine can be summarised as follows: fair healthcare assistance, continuity of treatment and constant monitoring, containment of costs, the possibility of developing businesses operating in the new technologies.

Telemedicine allows constant monitoring of the vital parameters of people at risk or those with diabetes or cardiovascular diseases, for example; the diagnosis process can be conducted in depth and the findings assessed in the GP's surgery, the pharmacy or the patient's home. A combination of telemedicine and artificial intelligence enables therapeutic choices to be made on the basis of the prognosis and can be used during therapeutic and rehabilitation pathways.

[101] Health Ministry, *Telemedicine, National guidelines*, 2014 page 10.

6.9 Social media and WhatsApp

Underpinning the logic of all social media lies the concept of interaction. Social media are an audience, not simply virtual, of millions of users who share ideas and thoughts on issues of all kinds: from current events to politics, from culture to sport, from cuisine to health.

The potential of these instruments is immediately clear: today 3.4 billion people access the Internet, with penetration of the total global population of 46% (in 2015, it was 42%); accounts activated on the social channels have exceeded 2 billion.

The number of people who access social media from mobile devices has seen the greatest growth: +17% (equal to 282 million people in the last year). The trends in the use of social platforms are very interesting: Facebook, with 1.5 billion active users is the social channel most used, by a long way. Services connected to instant messaging are also growing strongly, as shown by the 900 million active users on the WhatsApp platform, 800 million on Facebook Messenger and 200 million on Snapchat[102].

As stated previously, the issues of wellness, health and general medicine are among the group of subjects most covered on the Internet. Thus, we must ask ourselves what the role of the pharmacist can be in this context.

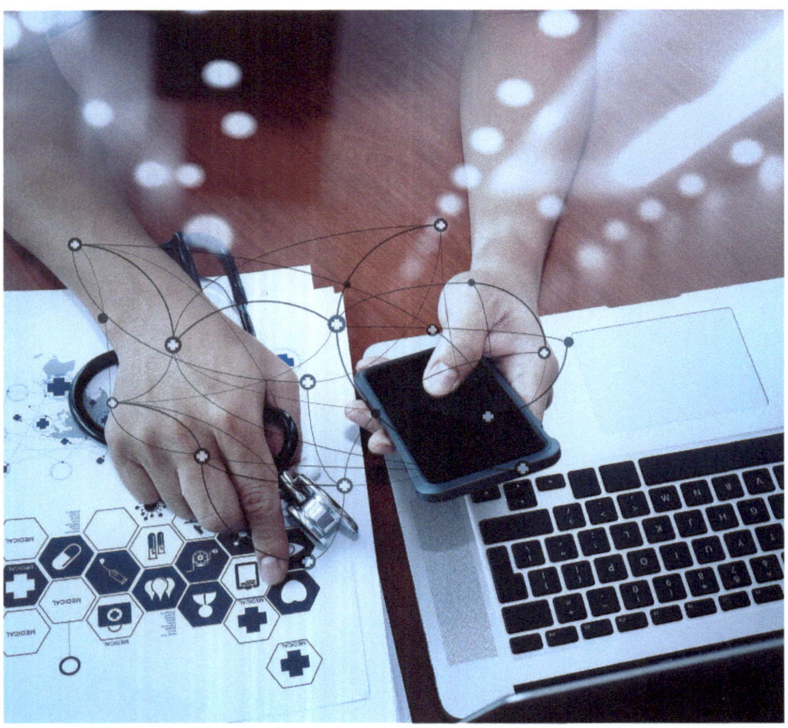

Facebook and the other social networks would allow health professionals to overcome the physical barrier represented by the walls of the pharmacy or clinic in order to reach their clients through a familiar instrument close to the users offering: consultation, advice on health protection and general information, obtaining in exchange personalised interaction for their users through "likes", sharing and comments.

The instant messaging services are a more direct and simple communication channel. By activating this instrument, district pharmacies can reach their clients rapidly and cheaply. Following the

[102] Digital in 2016, *We are social,* 28 January 2016.

example of a number of pharmacies that organised an original service of booking products and services in a simple and speedy way through WhatsApp, it will possible to be in direct contact with the pharmacy through a smartphone. By forwarding a request online, the user can immediately find out when to pick up the products after having checked their availability, avoiding queues and wasting time.

To obtain good results, a certain amount of training in the use of these social instruments is necessary.

In particular, it will be appropriate to be able to monitor the results for the purpose of planning efficient and targeted campaigns, always remembering that "The great difference of social media compared to traditional instruments lies in the fact that, with social information, an explicit interest is created that is self-perpetuated at the time of the interaction"[103] and therefore the use of these digital platforms automatically implies a change in the relationship with the patient/consumer for which it is necessary to be prepared.

[103] Fornaro A. 2014, http://www.safar.it/social-media-e-farmacia-quali-opportunita.

6.10 An App for smartphones and tablets

We now know that at least 40% of users at the global level access the Internet by means of a mobile device. This figure, constantly growing, has enabled the development and dissemination of a great number of applications linked to the world of wellness, health and healthcare assistance. There are 106 start-ups linked to artificial intelligence recently created in the health sector.

Given a similar plethora of initiatives, any example would only be partial, so we look at some of the most significant ones.

Some years ago, Apple launched its Research Kit with 5 mHealth Apps dedicated to Parkinson's disease, diabetes, cardiovascular diseases, asthma and breast cancer, which were mainly developed by research institutes; and others soon followed. The idea is to transform the more than 700 million iPhones into instruments in support of medical diagnosis. Many pharmacological research initiatives are already beginning to exploit mHealth technologies for clinical trials. Using smartphones with powerful processors and advanced sensors, movements can be tracked, measurements taken and very useful information recorded in pre- and post-marketing studies that make it possible to take part in clinical trials more easily and in a less invasive way. An mHealth App has the potential to involve an unprecedented number of individuals covering large geographical areas. According to Apple, the Research Kit will be a "research laboratory in the real world" and the data can be collected every second, remotely and throughout the world.

Another two Apps that are certainly interesting in the Italian panorama are Carepy, created by Carepysrl, and Pharmawizard developed by Datawizard. The first, created from an idea by three young computer scientists, is a system consisting of a mobile application and a software application installed on the pharmacies' terminal. Its creators define it as "the intelligent medicines box" because, on the one hand, it enables the user to display and organise their personal therapies and, on the other hand, places technology at the service of the pharmacist.

Pharmacists, after installing the Carepy platform in their pharmacy and inserting the patient's medicines by means of an optical scanner, can automatically manage their client, checking their supplies of medicines and overseeing the treatment, as well as sending targeted advice and suggestions.

This powerful tool also allows the pharmacies to consult product sales and consumption statistics in real time.

The App is potentially of great benefit for patients and anyone who possesses a smartphone can automatically receive specific indications on when to take the medicines.

Pharmawizard is a mobile App that enables the user to access information on medicines of concern to them, compare medicines with others, find equivalent alternatives, check any interactions and also simply find out the price of the medicine. All the data processed by Pharmawizard are taken directly from Farmadati's Medicines Database.

The webapp Codifa is an innovative example of an artificial intelligence application that makes information available on a mobile device. In addition to the availability of complete information on medicines and parapharmaceutical products, it offers a simple and advanced tool for immediately identifying the presence and severity of interactions among several medicines[104] and a system to support the prescription that demonstrates to the professional, in a few simple steps, all the various possible treatments, suggesting the most suitable for the specific patient.

The webapp also provides useful information to the patient for improved management of a specific treatment.

[104] The collaboration with the Department of Pharmacological and Biomolecular Sciences of Milan University, thanks to a team of experts coordinated by Prof. Racagni and Prof. Di Luca enables Codifa to use very accurate and detailed information on the interaction between medicines, foods and plant substances.

6.11 The new technologies: robots and virtual shelves

The word robot refers to any machine able to carry out work, more or less independently, in place of a human. According to some research carried out by SIRI – the Italian Association of Robotics and Automation – there could be around one and a half million robot units in the world, with an average annual growth of 9%[105].

Robots for the automation of the pharmacy include mechanical units made up of rollers, mechanical arms and housings that, operating synchronously, enable one of the main processes to be automated: the storage and handling of medicines and products to and from the storeroom. Many pharmacies choose to install a robot in order to save space and make better use of the display areas; others choose it to speed up and rationalise the loading and order management processes.

Virtual touch shelves are an innovative information tool that can be installed in district pharmacies and made available to the public. The function of virtual shelves is to represent certain products and services on a large screen through static or multimedia content – precisely as if they were actually on a real shelf – that can be changed in a matter of a few minutes or seconds, complete with all the features of interest to the consumer, such as the technical sheet, the price and any promotions. The touch screen monitors allow the public to navigate through the virtual shelves and to make choices in complete autonomy, where allowed by the OTC regulations.

[105] Appendino D., Vice President SIRI, *"I robot nel mondo"* (*Robots in the world*), 13 May 2016.

6.12 The international context

There are many examples of innovation in pharmacies, including in the international sphere. In the United Kingdom, the role of the pharmacist has been redefined under "Prescription for excellence", tending towards a more clinical profile. The pharmacist is involved in the initial choice of medicines and the subsequent monitoring of long-term prescriptions as well as adjustment of the dose during the treatment. The pharmacist is considered as a "general practice clinical pharmacist". A personal pharmacist is also envisaged, that is, a professional with whom a patient, choosing from a public list, can decide to register without implying a rigid constraint on only using that pharmacy. Thanks to the Medicines Reconciliation scheme, it is envisaged that "as soon as possible after the discharge of a patient, a discharge letter is sent to the family doctor and district pharmacist, appointed as the person responsible for the pharmaceutical treatments for that patient".

In Belgium, citizens can book a private visit with their pharmacist, who arranges a consultation in an area set up to ensure the necessary confidentiality. The service is aimed at patients with chronic conditions; a visit lasts for at least 15 minutes and the aim is to clarify any doubts about the way the medicines should be taken.

The consultation is then repeated every three months to evaluate progress and, at the same time, test the effectiveness of the previous meetings. The agreement signed by the Belgian pharmacies and the health services envisages financing whereby the owners receive € 20 per consultation in exchange for an improvement in adherence to the treatment, and therefore less need for access to the local medical facilities and hospitals, which are, of course, more costly.

In Japan, there are two main types of pharmacy. The first is the classic drugstore, a facility that can be part of a commercial retail sales business. This type of activity offers services on basic medicine, as well as parapharmaceutical products. The second type is the "dispensing pharmacy", generally located near a clinic or a hospital. In this type of pharmacy, the products are prepared in the laboratory, after which the client presents the prescription issued by their doctor. After packaging the medicine, the pharmacist explains to the client how to follow the treatment correctly.

In this context, KTX archiLAB has designed a new futuristic concept of the Japanese pharmacy. In Japan, the idea of a cure is associated with natural elements that convey the idea of peace and serenity: inside buildings, there are natural materials such as trees, flowers and walls, all associated with innovative design elements. Pharmacies are located on major streets, the external facade has sharp corners, while most interiors have minimal decor.

The straight, clean lines enriched with openings through which light enters indirectly give the feeling of order, clarity and peace; in this way, an attempt is made to reinforce the psychological elements that are required and that the patient expects to see during the course of the treatment.

Traditionally, the patient sends or delivers a prescription to the reception desk and, while the pharmacist prepares the personalised medicines in the laboratory, the patient sits in the waiting room surrounded by the interior architecture as described above. Once the medicines are ready, the patient is called back to reception or is joined by the pharmacist in the waiting area to receive detailed explanations about the prescription.

These "little" touches can make a big difference, providing an image of high-quality service and improving the results of the therapy.

6.13 Innovations in the United States

The innovations promoted in the United States deserve a fuller discussion. Here, we present the following:

I. The PillPack case
II. The 3D tablet printing process
III. IBM Watson
IV. The Walgreens & Duane Reade case
V. The PatientsLikeMe case

I The PillPack case

PillPack is simply a revolutionary pharmacy, which has changed the management of the pharmacological system for more than 32 million people, who each take more than five medicines every month. The service involves the delivery of the pharmacological treatment, differing according to the specific patient, pre-packaged in single-use, single-dose bags in a practical dispenser, indicating the time and day they are to be taken. First, the quantity and type of medicines to be taken as prescribed by the doctor are communicated to the PillPack company by the pharmacist, along with the patient's health insurance information. By means of the distribution chain, the company send the treatment required to the pharmacy chosen by the patient (which the patient can change at any time) every 15 days. The service is accompanied by a notification via email and/or SMS that reminds the patient when to pick up the medicines and, if required, how and when to take them every day.
Thanks to PillPack, the patients manage their own pharmacological treatment in the simplest way, they no longer forget when to take a medicine because, using the dispenser, the treatment is delivered regularly. In addition, the patient can consult their bills online, where the costs of the medicines are given, showing the costs that are reimbursed and those that are not.

II The 3D tablet printing process

Another area of interest is 3D printing. The process of 3D printing is the creation of three-dimensional objects by means of additive production, starting from a 3D digital model. The digital model is produced with dedicated software and subsequently processed before being created, layer by layer, by a 3D printer. This new technology could potentially change the way in which we take medicines or even their kinetics in the human body in the coming decade. Thanks to 3D printing technology, an innovative method of turning active ingredients into tablets will be possible. MakerBot Replicator, the innovator of the technology that enables 3D printing of pharmaceutical tablets in specific geometric shapes and sizes, argues that the change of pharmacokinetics (and therefore the pharmacodynamic effects) can become an important driver in the production of medicines with great potential for the patient. Researchers who first conducted tests in this area produced tablets in various forms, such as pyramids, cubes and spheres, perfectly equal in composition and final volume. Underpinning the research was the discovery that the area/volume ratio can be a determining property in the kinetics of the release of the medicine. In the light of the fact that some patients require medicines that act more quickly, while others need medicines that are released more gradually over a longer period of time, 3D printing offers the possibility of personalising identical active ingredients for the individual needs of the patients. If the potential of these new technologies is confirmed, it will be possible in the near future to proceed directly with the printing of medicines at home and this will undoubtedly produce cost benefits in addition to ensuring access to treatments for persons with poor mobility and in urgent situations.
However, there is a need to be aware of some problems, such as self-production of medicines or narcotics and the risk of being attacked by hackers who could spread viruses and malware in the networks of technological systems.

III IBM Watson

IBM scientists have created a cognitive super-computer that understands natural human language and is able to respond to questions of all kinds, providing precise and accurate answers. It was developed by the IBM team led by David Ferrucci as part of the "DeepQA" project and the name was chosen in honour of the first president of IBM, Thomas J. Watson.
Watson is capable of doing much more than search engines such as Google and Bing, always finding the most probabilistically correct answer. IBM's general consultant, Robert

C. Weber, proposed the use of Watson in legal research; the company intends to use Watson where there is a vast amount of unstructured information that makes the decision-making process complex and elaborate, such as in telecommunications, financial services and government decisions. IBM is also considering launching the DeepQA application on the market. Currently, the price would exceed a million dollars but, thanks to technological improvements, IBM expects this to fall within a decade.
In the health sphere, medical personnel can be provided with much support in clinical decisions, using Watson's natural language, with its ability to generate hypotheses and its capacity for evidence-based learning. Watson is a kind of super-doctor, which can help in the treatment of patients following a series of steps: it receives a question in which the symptoms and other correlated factors are specified and then the most important components are extracted from the information in order to process them with the patients' data, seeking possible correlations in their clinical history; thereafter, it examines the data available from other sources to formulate and test hypotheses and, finally, it provides a list of recommendations identified and classified by level of evidence. The data sources that Watson uses are multiple and range from treatment guidelines to electronic medical records, annotations of specialist doctors and nurses, research materials, clinical trials, magazine articles and information about the patient. Watson has demonstrated a capacity to discover previously unknown connections between diseases, succeeding in changing the indications on the basis of new information.
Johnson & Johnson is collaborating with the IBM Watson Discovery Advisor team in order to teach Watson to read and understand scientific articles and interpret the results of clinical trials in order to develop and evaluate medicines and other treatments. In addition, Sanofi is exploring how it can accelerate the discovery of alternative indications for existing medicines.

IV The Walgreens & Duane Reade case

The Walgreens Company is the largest chain of US pharmacies, founded in Chicago in 1901; today it represents an original format created from a combination of drugstore, convenience shop, pharmacy and parapharmacy, and is regarded as an institution in America because often these commercial businesses are also health assistance centres open 24/7. Duane Reade is also a forerunner of this model, also in the United States and also part of the Walgreen Boots Alliance (WBA). Opened in the 1960s in New York, it was based on a very innovative concept for those days: dividing the display space into separate but complementary areas for wellness and health, such as, for example, a "food" zone for products to take away or consume in the bar/restaurant; household goods and small appliances, a cosmetics area (hairdresser, nail parlour, make-up, etc.); a pharmacy/parapharmacy and a doctor's surgery, always open.

WBA is the leading global group in health, pharmacies and wellness, the explicit aim of which is to improve people's lifestyles. This was a very courageous undertaking given that Walgreens Boots Alliance is a young company, which, as we know it today, was created through a merger between Walgreens and Alliance Boots in December 2014. Thanks to this merger, two leading companies, for a long time icons in the distribution of health services, were combined into a single brand. Some data may be indicative of the importance of the brand; currently, it has more than 13,200 sales outlets in the world, almost entirely pharmacies, 390 distribution centres divided between Europe and the United States with a single partner and 400,000 employees from 25 countries. In northern Europe, Boots Alliance has 2845 sales outlets, a network of 6000 Alphega pharmacies and a wholesale distribution chain with 110 centres.

The creation of Walgreens Boots Alliance has become synonymous with a global and integrated platform able to provide innovative ways of tackling the challenges on matters of health and wellness, in all situations. The examples concerning the following phases of the treatment chain are representative: treatment in the acute phase, treatment and monitoring of chronic conditions, health and general wellness.

As regards innovations in the acute phases, the following are significant:

- pharyngeal swabs;
- screening for moles.

Of itself, the pharyngeal swab does not constitute an innovation; for some time, this diagnostic examination has been used to determine the pathogenic agent responsible for a disease; the innovation lies in having brought this type of examination to the pharmacy, as the case from the United Kingdom demonstrates. Thanks to efficient coordination with the National Health Service, it has been possible to spread the service to local pharmacies and disseminate this practice among a growing number of individuals, leading to an overall reduction in the costs. By recognising the pathogenic agent with greater accuracy, it has been possible to prescribe antibiotics only when necessary, an absolutely necessary step in combatting the increasingly looming threat of antibiotic resistance on a global scale and allowing the burden of work to be lightened for doctors and making best use of the resources available.

Teledermatology in the pharmacy is a way of disseminating good practices in preventing skin cancer. This type of screening, carried out in pharmacies, has had a positive impact,

especially in northern Europe, an area where the percentage of people with melanoma is increasing due to the duration of exposure to sunlight and the lack of pigmentation in the skin of its inhabitants. Thanks to new technologies, the pharmacy has become the most suitable place where the patient can tackle this often neglected problem. Screening allows macroscopic and dermoscopic images to be collected and compared in a database of sample images, detecting any type of anomaly, which is then transmitted to specialist dermatologists for additional tests.
In analysing the innovations that can be introduced for the treatment and monitoring of chronic conditions, it is important to underline that the contribution of the pharmacy can be significant if, and only if, it is integrated with the rest of the health system, irrespective of the public or private nature of the payers. Thanks to the new technologies, the pharmacy assumes a role of primary importance in screening, diagnostics, adherence to treatment by the patients, research and precision medicine.

The data gathered at every stage must be transmitted in an unequivocal way to the rest of the health system to enable progressive reduction of the costs that have an impact on the treatment of chronic conditions.
Screening and diagnostics, in addition to detecting symptoms of diseases in the acute phase, leads to early detection of these diseases, thereby reducing the mortality associated with them. Through practices of therapeutic adherence, working jointly with the NHS, pharmacies also take on a fundamental role in the patient's journey, along with considerable reduction in costs for the health system.
Precision medicine, by reconnecting with the fundamental issue of therapeutic adherence, enables the right treatments to be provided in the right dosage and at the most appropriate time.
In conclusion, with regard to health and general wellness, the Walgreens Boots Alliance group is demonstrating that pharmacies can take on the task of incentivising and disseminating healthy and virtuous behaviours, such as walking, measuring blood pressure, taking drugs and medicines at the most appropriate times.
To further improve this aspect, a system of scoring is being studied that enables patients to be incentivised to achieve established objectives. A great contribution to this system of rewards will be provided by digital technologies that allow dialogue to be established between pharmacists, patients and the rest of the health system.
In some countries, such as the United Kingdom, Ireland, Portugal, Finland, the United States, Canada, Australia, New Zealand and in some Swiss Cantons and French regions, one of the major innovations has been the introduction of the possibility of carrying out vaccinations

in pharmacies. If other countries want to follow suit, communication campaigns will be necessary to spread the added value of this practice, in order to avoid introducing this activity in the pharmacies as just another service added to an existing list.
All these innovations can function if designed and spread in a collaborative way with the rest of the health system, allowing all the actors involved to best deliver their professionalism and experience.

V The PatientsLikeMe case

PatientsLikeMe is an American association founded in 2004 by two brothers, Jamie and Ben Heywood. It is privately financed and dedicated to improving the quality of life of people who have been diagnosed with a "life-changing" disease.
PatientsLikeMe was inspired by the life experience of Stephen Heywood who, at the age of 29, was diagnosed with a form of amyotrophic lateral sclerosis (ALS) or Lou Gehrig's disease. After the diagnosis of ALS, Stephen's family founded a non-profit organisation, the ALS Therapy Development Institute, in an attempt to slow down his disease and treat its symptoms.

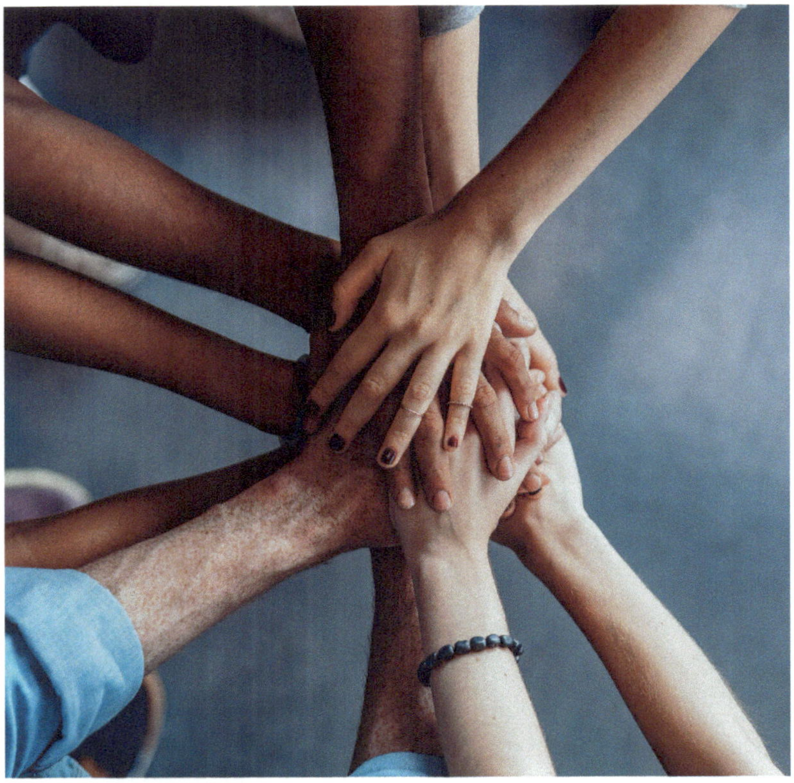

Like Stephen, other patients in the world are experiencing the same situation, asking themselves many questions on their state of health and what they can do, from the pharmacological point of view and otherwise, in order to improve it. On this premise, PatientsLikeMe was created, a network and, at the same time, a research platform. A community of patients, doctors and organisations was established to inform, assist and make people suffering from debilitating disease more aware, guaranteeing them access to the information and services required for the management of their disease. Through the network, patients and

their families can remain in contact with other patients with the same disease and share their respective experiences. The PatientsLikeMe website is a social network made up of patients along the lines of the model of user-generated content sites.
Users have the possibility of learning from the aggregate data and seeing what type of treatment other patients are undertaking. Registration on the site is free of charge and involves the collection of personal data, with a detailed explanation of how the data are used and an appropriate disclaimer on the privacy policy adopted.
Registered users can create their own profile and a personal area, managing the information they want to make public or not. Members of the site use social instruments like forums, private messages and updated profiles.
PatientsLikeMe is a support mechanism that contributes to improving the management and control of diseases. With almost 500,000 members, PatientsLikeMe is a reliable source of information on diseases and has enabled the publication of more than 80 research studies of excellent quality.

Conclusions[106]

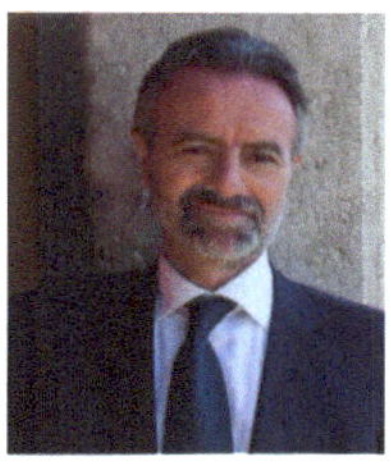

Luca Pani

The governance of the medicines of the future, which will enable the entire pharmaceutical chain to be truly resilient, will be based on certain, very solid principles.

The example that we have just given of PatientsLikeMe, an online network open to all (patients and families) where information on their health can be registered in a secure way and they can connect with other individuals with the same disease, or others, demonstrates how a contribution to clinical research can be made even from home.

Thanks to the American partnership with Walgreens, PatientsLikeMe share their experience of medicines and so provide information, and not only data, on medicines that they use, which then becomes an incredible source of knowledge. We live in a global system that moves very rapidly; we can debate forever whether this is right or not but, in the meantime, we must be able to help the consumers/patients wherever they are in such a way that the control of their health is no further away than the distance between them and their mobile phone.

Monitoring of this new consumer/patient and all the follow-ups through an App, social media and Web platforms will therefore require a very close and personal dialogue between all healthcare operators who are concerned with the sick or, even better, healthy individuals at risk. But that will not be enough. As has been amply demonstrated by the controversy over vaccines that has swept through the entire world, another issue is the education campaigns and preventive health actions that must take account of the emotions that lie beneath certain choices.

Taking account of patients' needs means fully recognising their transformation into consumers. In trying to find out whether a product/service will do the job and, as we have seen, leaving behind the paternalistic model, we must encourage patients to contribute the data that concerns what we do. Requesting feedback can produce unexpected answers and, for those who are truly interested in what others think, adjustments in the organisation of the work and the "room for action", changing its presentation and structure, in some way favouring the products or services that are most appreciated and sought after and abandoning the others.

These considerations form part of the general concept at the basis of the most modern digital marketing that, which is above all, individualised and made to measure for each individual; priorities should not be defined from above and we should not take for granted that a communication strategy that works for all will also work for each individual.

[106] Reworked by; Pani L., editorials of *The Blind Spot/Il Punto Cieco*, Punto Effe, LSWR-EDRA, 2017, Milan.

Thanks to the diabolical and precise profiling based on the so-called cookies, by now we are used to the fact that, when we go to a product site (whatever it may be), we are automatically presented with what we will most probably like. It often works precisely because, having ourselves given permission for the of cookies, we have authorised our navigation patterns and our past choices to be studied, and the series of all the choices already made by a population of millions of users who navigate that site predict those of the future. Why should this not also apply to medicines?

In practice, it is as if we are shaping the market that we wish to find in a continuous and dynamic way. Think what could happen if, in the same way as has happened with TripAdvisor for hotels and Zagat for restaurants, consumers/patients could immediately transmit their experience and satisfaction (number of stars) online concerning services regarding their health. It is a sure bet that the highest scores will be given to those facilities that "react" rapidly to requests and will depend on their capacity to interact in a personalised way in the field of information technology. But it is logical to assume that all this will not be free of charge. The costs to be faced will come from the need to invest in new IT tools, in algorithms and dedicated software concerned mainly with customer relationship management, a discipline that – in brief – concerns all those practices, strategies and technologies that companies use for managing, and above all analysing, interactions between consumers and data through the evaluation of their lifestyles that currently – and it is very relevant for those in the health professions – are easily measurable, portable and important for the diagnosis, therapy and prognosis of pharmacological treatments.

Pharmaceutical resilience will also be seen in the need to invest in the personalisation of services oriented to the consumer/patient and will have at least three main centres of investment that, in the medium to long term, could lead to better use of resources:

- Improvement of the attractiveness (including aesthetic) of IT services through a noticeable and measurable level of their quality. The use of IT serves to reinforce the positive perception of the quality of the service delivered but its personalisation makes it, if so desired, individual and traceable with absolute certainty at the level of the individual, allowing remuneration for the capacity, for example, of certain programmes (Apps or Web platforms) to proactively avoid suspension of a necessary therapy or the use of inadequate treatments.

- The costs that can be saved by the suspension of unnecessary actions amount to up to 30% in other industries and, in healthcare assistance, the early identification both of diseases and the most appropriate treatments demonstrate the enormous value in the medium and long term, not only economically but also on the psychological level and in terms of side effects (lack of efficacy and adverse reactions). Moreover, in accordance with common experience and that of various academics, the greater need for this type of service is with those patients who use the most costly medicines (for example, in hospitals). Saving costs through certification of the suspension of unnecessary actions translates into certifiably avoided costs.

- An increase in the so-called economies of scope, more correctly known as "economies of diversification" or even "economies of range" that produce savings thanks to the joint production of different products or by pursuing different objectives with the same production factors (the same resources, the same structures and the same know-how). The economies of range are probably the most interesting because they are based on the theory that when a consumer/patient is loyal to the services, those who provide them can broaden them with a series of other services (for example, screening) at very competitive market prices, because they can rely on a stable and continuous income.

If, therefore, ICT will also be required to analyse the information flows and the associated (or avoidable) costs with the lifestyles of consumers/patients, then the preeminent issue will be to understand how to certify this enormous mass of data and, above all, for what purpose. In the current socio-economic context, two primary objectives emerge: precision medicine and healthcare assistance targeted at the individual patient who, contrary to what may be thought, is not homogeneous, either in identity or nature. Although everyone knows by now that precision medicine is made up of the 4 Ps – Personalisation, Prevention, Prediction and Participation – few realise that the end of the paternalistic model and the emergence of individual and collective participation will permanently transform the very structure of biology and medicine, making them ipso facto information sciences. At this point, the flow of certified data and their analysis, be they structured or otherwise, will have to be used to "tailor-make" healthcare assistance worthy of the name for every individual patient, not only on the basis of the sequencing of their DNA but also with regard to organisational, social and psychological appropriateness. All the individuals who go to a doctor or enter a pharmacy also enter a network to be navigated, without a helmsman and in a sea of uncontrollable data that represents everything and the opposite of everything. The ability to transform this possibility of access to information into the competitive advantage of knowledge depends on our capacity to accept the change and anticipate it in an innovative way. The future will not sit and wait for us for long.
What are the limits of what we have related in these editorials in the last year? Certainly, they reflect, even though on the basis of the data in the current literature, my own personal

vision of what I believe is important in what is happening in the interface between biology, medicine and information technology, whatever these three nouns now define. The second point derives from my hypothesis that the massive use of the Internet will render obsolete, de facto non-existent, not only the borders between many countries (what we define with an all-inclusive and therefore equally pointless name "the Global world!") but also those between the various roles.
We not only find ourselves in the midst of a paradigm shift but in the midst of a series of continuous paradigm shifts (paradigm shocks) that will change our way of practising all the professions that are concerned, at any level, with human health. And not only those. The other limit is that intrinsic to the editorial structure of these pages that necessitated, within a finite and short number of characters, some points for reflection that could not be explored as much in depth as they deserved. It is difficult in these cases, even more so when speaking and writing about healthcare assistance, to maintain a neutral and objective point of view when describing general principles that must necessarily be corrected by the various realities in which they are applied.
This "paradigm shock" shifts rapidly and leads us to mysterious places.

What has the virtual money Bitcoin, for example, to do with the way in which we take care of our health in order to live much longer and better? Blockchain technology (translated clumsily in Italian as Catena a Blocchi or Blocchi Concatenati) at the basis of Bitcoin is already considered the new, and currently the only paradigm by which to share network data bringing another level of security and, above all, productivity, to the digital world. A blockchain is a form of distributed database made up of packets of data recorded digitally (a block) that cannot be modified because they are stored in a linear chain to which a string of encrypted and unique codes is assigned. The beauty of this technology is that it is based on decentralised procedures where every device that takes part in the chain stores inside it an identical copy of the same blocks, which also cannot be modified. It can immediately be understood how this chain could be crucial for storing sensitive information such as data concerning our health.
At the end of 2016, when I began to speak on various occasions with Richard Etwaru (Chief Digital Health Officer of IMS-Quintiles), William King (CEO of Zephyr Health) and Giorgio Albonetti (Chairman of EDRA-LSWR) about the opportunity to use this technology to encrypt sensitive data concerning our health, it seemed that there would be a long time to wait to solve a series of technical problems to perfect it. Less than a year later, the possibility of this happening is no longer so remote, for at least three reasons. Firstly, the discussion on Big Data will be able to stop dealing endlessly with the famous 4 Vs (Volume, Velocity, Variety

and Veracity) and tackle the only real elephant in the room, that is, security. Secondly, it is remarkable that the application of Blockchain to health data will manage to bring together the last two bulwarks of true democracy: disease and information technology. The solidity and controlled access to certified sensitive data of every one of us are two pillars around which the challenge of all health systems revolves. Whoever succeeds in certifying the identity of each one of us, with biometric certainty and in a way no longer open to modification, will not even have to ask our name. The Inpeco Corporation[107] is not far from achieving this, which is at the basis of what is defined as total patient management (TPM). From that moment on, sharing will also make health data more reliable for subsequent processing and the ownership of the individual block on the user's device will allow others to take part in this sharing, which can always be revoked on an individual basis.
This aspect, in my opinion, is the most important of all because, if certain technical problems are solved, Blockchain really seems to be the solution to constructing immense health databases in a universally accessible way, removing the risks and extending the opportunities, including predictive, that will be derived from their intelligent analysis. In this way, the volume of data will acquire value and we will finally move from the Internet of Things to the Internet of Value. Only in this way will widespread, granular and detailed information finally become new knowledge, something that more than 20 years of mass Internet use have not managed to achieve.

[107] www.inpeco.com.